Fontana A–Z of Dog Care

D0040461

Stephen Schneck is a novelist, journalist and the sole support of two cats and a dog. A conscientious pet owner, he wanted to know more about his pets' health, but could not find any book on practical home medical treatment for them. So he decided to write one. Requiring expert advice, he went to an expert . . .

Nigel Norris, BVSc, MRCVS, who qualified from the University of Bristol in 1965 and has been a practising veterinarian in London for many years.

Fontana A-Z of
Dog Care

Stephen Schneck
with Nigel Norris BVSC MRCVS

Introduction by Henry Carter
Past President, British Small Animal
Veterinary Association

FONTANA/COLLINS

To my Son Matthew

Acknowledgments

M.D. Corner, B Vet Med, MRCVS
Dr P.G.C. Bedford, PhD, B Vet Med,
MRCVS
and Caroline

First published by William Collins Sons
& Co Ltd, 1975
First issued in Fontana 1979

Made and printed in Great Britain by
Richard Clay (The Chaucer Press) Ltd,
Bungay, Suffolk

Introduction

One of the many problems facing veterinary surgeons is how to explain, in non-technical language, what is wrong with a pet animal so that the owner can understand and, if possible, help the healing process. The layman can only be expected to have a superficial knowledge of anatomy and physiology, and the rapid advances in diagnosis and treatment in recent years have made the gulf between professional adviser and client even wider.

Veterinarians in small-animal practice soon gain experience in explaining, as simply as possible, what may be a very complex condition. Nevertheless, most of us have felt the need for an up-to-date book compiled especially for the pet owner. *Collins A to Z of Dog Care*, written by a pet owner in collaboration with a practising veterinary surgeon, neatly fills this gap. Factually correct, the information is presented in clear everyday language which will give useful guidance to even the most inexperienced owner with little or no knowledge of biology.

In many parts of the world, a dog owner may be far from the nearest veterinarian, and though in some countries flying doctor services are available, the 'flying vet' is, as yet, a luxury pet owners cannot afford. In these remote areas antibiotics and other medicines are available, but they are of little use without some knowledge and advice on how to use them. In the United Kingdom, and in many other countries, antibiotics etc. are (quite rightly) available only on the prescription of a member of the veterinary profession. There are, however, many simple and effective remedies which can be used before professional advice is sought or when it is not possible to get immediate treatment from a vet.

This book helps the owner cope with both situations and also gives the basic rules for prompt and effective first aid in emergencies.

The British Small Animal Veterinary Association, representing veterinary surgeons not only in the UK but all over the world, is most concerned that people should look after their pets in a responsible way. This means caring for the health and welfare of the animal and being alert for any changes which may be signs of impending illness. *Collins A to Z of Dog Care* should be of considerable help in furthering this aim and will, I am sure, be welcomed by both pet owners and veterinary surgeons.

Henry Carter MRCVS
Past President British Small Animal
Veterinary Association

How to use this book

The main entries are arranged alphabetically for quick and easy reference, and within each entry the information is given in a logical sequence of causes, symptoms or description, and treatment, where applicable, to make the process of diagnosing and treating any condition as simple and speedy as possible. For instance, if your dog has a nosebleed, just look up the entry on 'Nosebleed', and follow the instructions for treatment.

If the condition is a more complex one, and you are not exactly sure what it is, you may wish to consult the index at the beginning of the book. Information is indexed in three ways: under the disease name, under the part of the body affected, and under major symptoms displayed. For example, slipped disc is indexed under 'S' and 'D', as would be expected, but also under 'Back' and 'Pain in the back'. So if you observe that your dog is suffering from pain in the back, but don't know what is wrong, you can easily find out a possible cause by looking up either 'Back' or 'Pain in the back'. Check to see if the related symptoms described in the entry are present in your dog, thus confirming the condition.

Index

A

worms, 1

Abnormal vaginal discharge, 130

Abortion, 2, 87; see also Mating; Mismating (mésalliance)

Abrasions, 34, 63

Abscesses: 3, 20, 24, 47
of the anal glands, 3, 47
of the ano-rectal passage, 47
of tooth-roots, 3
pointing of, 3
specific, 3
swelling of, 3

Absence of tear ducts, 150

Accidental overdose of insulin, see Poisoning (insulin)

Accidents: 8, 23, 25, 26, 30, 39, 53, 69, 73, 78, 92, 99, 101, 144, 166
car, 8, 30, 39, 53, 166
road, 69, 99, 101
with fish-hooks, 73

Acetone-smelling breath, 55; and see Diabetes

Acid burns, 35, 129

Acid poisoning, see Poisoning

Acquired deafness, see Deafness

Acute abdomen, 169

Acute eczema, 63

Acute eczema, moist, 63

Acute form of canine virus hepatitis, see Canine virus hepatitis

Acute kidney failure, 129

Acute middle ear infection: 4
loss of balance, 4

Acute otitis: 5, 77; see also Ear mites; Middle ear infection
acute itching, 5
acute soreness, 5
severe inflammation, 5

Agalactia: 96, 124

Abdomen:
acute, 169
distension of the, 28, 167
enlargement of the, 70, 153
fluid in the, 153, 172
injuries to the, 99
intestines protruding from the, 99
pain in the, 22, 81, 92, 125, 129, 167
rigidity of the, 147
rupture of the, see Hernia
soreness of the, 107
swelling of the, 28, 136, 153
tenseness of the, 147

Abdominal enlargement, 70, 153

Abdominal pain: 22, 81, 125, 129, 167
front legs extended, 81
rear legs extended, 81
restlessness, 81, 125
seeking out cold places to lie on, 81, 125

Abdominal tumours, 14, 153, 172

Ability to detect vibrations, 51

Abnormal bowel movement: 1, 47, 56, 133
blood in faeces, 1
colour, 1
constipation, 1, 133
diarrhoea, 1, 56
flattened or ribbon-like faeces, 1, 133
hard and soft stool, 1
odour, 1
pain, 47, 133
quantity, 1
unusual object in faeces, 1

at birth of first litter, 96
restless behaviour of puppies, 96

Aimless wandering, 60

Air sickness, see Motion sickness

Alkali burns, see Burns

Alkali poisoning, see Poisoning

Allergic asthma: 6
chestiness, 6
short-windedness, 6
wheeziness, 6

Allergic dermatitis: 6
intense itching, 6
intense scratching, 6
red patches, sore, 6
red patches, weeping, 6

Allergies: 6, 63
allergic asthma, 6
allergic dermatitis, 6
hay fever, 6
hives, 6
nettlerash, 6
of the respiratory tract, 6
of the skin, 6, 146

Allergies of the respiratory tract: 6
allergic asthma, 6
hay fever, 6

Allergies of the skin: 6, 146
allergic dermatitis, 6
hives, 6
nettlerash, 6

Alopecia, see Baldness

Amputation, 7

Anaemia: 8, 144
lethargy, 8
rapid pulse, 8
unnatural pallor around the eyes, gums, nose, 8

Anal adenoma, see Anal tumours

Anal eczema, 10, 63

Analgesics, 9

Anal gland abscesses, 3

Anal glands: 3, 10, 47
abscesses of the, 3, 47

swelling of the scrotum, 92
traumatic, 92
umbilical:
in puppies, 92
protrusion of intestinal fat, 92
Hiccups, **93**
High blood pressure, 121
High fever: 81, 135, 161, 164
dry coat, 81
dry, hot nose, 81
dull eyes, 81
worn expression, 81
High temperature, 37, 60, 91, 107, 127, 130, 162
Hind legs, 30, 61, 64, 78
Hip dysplasia, 29
Hip joint: 29, 59
dislocated, 59
false, development of a, 59
Hives: 6
raised patches on body, 6
swollen eyelids, 6
swollen face, 6
Hobbling, 77, 78
Hormonal imbalance, 63, 96, 146
Hormone deficiency, 89
Humans bitten by dogs, **94**
Hysteria: 39, **95**; and see Fits
barking, 95
involuntary passage of faeces and urine, 95
unresponsiveness to commands, 95

I

Impaction of large intestine, 67
Inability to breathe, 129
Inability to give milk, **96**, 124
Inability to pass urine, 167
Inability to stand or walk, 78; and see Fractures of the pelvis

Incised wounds, 174
Incoordination: 74, 78, 109, 114, 129
during fits, 74
induced by fractures of the skull, 78
Increased appetite, 14, 55
Increased body temperature, 68, 114, 160
Increased thirst, 55, 68, 107, 130, 136
Increased urination, 55
Increased weight, 172
Indigestion, 169
Infected teeth, 3, 16
Infected wounds, 20, 73, 80
Infection: 4, 5, 8, 13, 16, 18, 20, 23, 24, 28, 51, 68, 80, 81, 82, 86, 104, 148, 158
of the bowel, 28
of the ear, 24, 51
of the eye, 23
of the gums, 82, 158
of the intestines, 81
of the lungs, see Pneumonia
of the middle ear, 4, 24, 86
of the mouth, 82
of the stomach, 81
of the throat, 82
Infectious conditions of the eye, 46
Infectious diseases, 13, 160, 169
Infectious ringworm, 146
Infectious skin diseases, 146
Inflammation: 58, 63, 97, 112, 127, 169
of the ear, 112
of the gullet, 169
of the penis, 58
of the pleura, 127
of the skin, 63, 129
of the tongue, **97**
Inguinal canal, 92,
Inguinal hernia, see Hernia
Injections, **98**
Injuries: 18, 23, 39, 53, 78, 99, 110, 144, 174
to the abdomen, **99**
to the brain, 23
to the chest, 174
to the ears, 18
to the eyes, 18, 23

to the leg, 18
to the limbs, 78
to the paws, 110
Insensitivity to pain, 30
Insulin coma, 55
Insulin poisoning: 55, 129
collapse, 129
incoordination, 129
staggering, 129
unconsciousness, 129
Interdigital cyst, 84, **100**
Internal bleeding: 99, **101**, 129
cold paws, 101
pallor of mucous membranes, 101
pronounced weakness, 101
rapid but weak pulse rate, 101
Internal parasites, 172, 173
Intestinal obstruction, 169
Intestinal protrusion, 99
Intestines: 26, 81, 99
bleeding from the, 25, 26
infection of the, 81
protruding from the abdomen, 99
Involuntary passage of faeces and urine, 95; and see Fits; Hysteria
Iodine deficiency, 17
Iron deficiency, 8
Irregular heat periods, 136
Irretractable penis, **102**
Irritation of the ear: 108, 112
acute, 112
from lice, 108
Itching, 6, 17, 63
intense, 6
Itch-scratch cycle, 6; and see Skin

J

Jaundice, 37, 107, 129
Jaw: 42, 78
clicking of the, 42
fractures of the, 78

S

Safety pins, swallowing,
152
St Vitus' Dance, 42
Saline solution, **140**
Salivation, profuse, 74,
117, 129, 158
Sarcoptic mange, 112,
146
Scalds, **35**
Scratching: 6, 24, 63,
65, 77, 112
  constant, 63
  intense, 63
Screaming, 120
Scrotal hernia, see Hernia
Scrotum, swelling of the,
92
Scurf, see Dandruff
Sea sickness, see Motion
sickness
Season, see Mating
Sebaceous cyst, **141**
Sedative overdose, **142**
Self-mutilation, acci-
dental, 99
Sensation, loss of, 30
Severe abdominal pains,
167
Shaking the head, 74, 77,
112
Shampooing a dog, **143**
Shivering, 44, 164
Shock: 7, 8, 35, 39, 66,
87, 99, 101, 103, 109,
126, 129, **144**, 166, 174
  apathy, 144
  complete collapse, 144
  low body temperature,
  144
  pale gums, tongue, 144
  rapid, shallow breathing,
  144
  rapid, thready pulse, 144
  thirst, 144
Shortening (of fractured
limbs), 78
Short-windedness, 6
Signs of approaching
birth, see Birth
Simple fractures, 78
Sinus (small puncture
wound), 161
Sinuses, infection of the,
see Sinusitis
Sinusitis: 16, 44, 118, **145**

loss of appetite, 145
nasal discharge, 145
sneezing bouts, 145
skin:
  abrasions, 34
  abscesses, 3, 20
  allergic dermatitis, 6
  allergies, 6
  bedsores, 38
  boils, 3
  breaks in the, 84, 139
  bruises, 34
  calluses, 38
  capped elbow, 38
  carbuncles, 3
  crusts, 35, 112
  cuts, 25, 34, 105, 110
  dandruff, 52
  dry, 63, 81
  eczema, 63
  eruptions, 104
  flaking, 63, 64
  frostbite, 79
  hairlessness, 146
  inflamed patches on the,
  129
  itch-scratch cycle, 6
  lumps on the, 6
  mange, 112, 139, 146
  moist, 63
  nettlerash, 6
  patches, 6, 129, 139
  pustules, 84, 141
  redness, 6, 63, 79, 82
  ringworm, 129, 139
  scalds, 35
  scaling, 129
  scurf, 52
  sebaceous cyst, 141
  shiny, 77
  sores, 6
  swelling, 3, 79
  thickening, 38, 112
  warts, 170
  weeping, 6, 35
Skin conditions, 84, 146
Skin diseases: 65, 84, 112,
146
  allergies, 146
  contagious, 146
  hereditary, 146
  infectious, 146
  neuroses, 146
  non-contagious, 146
Skin eruptions, 104
Skin lesions, 63
Skin patches, 6
Skull, fractures of the: 78
  incoordination, 78
  nosebleeds, 78

unconsciousness, 78
Sleepiness, 161
Slipped disc, 30, 47, **147**
Slowness of movement,
107
Sneezing: 6, 145, **148**
  accompanied by nasal
  discharge, 148
  continual, 148
  intermittent, 148
  prolonged, 148
  strenuous, 148
Soft palate, prolonged, 29
Soft stool, 1
Sore abdomen, 107
Sore anus, 56, 85
Sore chest, 128
Sore eyes, 107
Sore mouth, 14
Sore nipples, 120
Sore pad, 71
Sore paws, 49
Sores, 6
Specific abscesses, 3
Spinal column, disloca-
tion of the, 30
Spleen, enlargement of
the, 153
Sprains, 45, 105, 110, **149**
Squeaking sounds, see
Ear
Staggering, 129, 170
Stains at the corner of the
eye, **150**
Stiffness, 52
Stings: 103, **151**
  bee, 151
  jelly-fish, 103
  wasp, 151
Stomach infection, 16,
81
Stomach, injuries to the,
see Injuries to the
abdomen
Stomach ulcer, 26
Stomatitis, 16
Stool: 1
  hard, 1
  loose, 1
  pain when passing, 1
Straining to pass a
motion, 47, 88
Strains, 45, 105, 149
Strangulation of the
bowel, 92
Strokes, 23, 166
Strychnine poisoning:
129
  convulsions, 129
  death, 129

1 Abnormal Bowel Movement

See also **Blood in Bowel Movement**

An abnormal bowel movement may be distinguished from a normal one by:

Texture
Hard (constipation).
Soft (diarrhoea).

Colour
Blood in faeces: see a vet – there could be ulcers or tumours.
Too pale: suspect problems with gall bladder or pancreas.
Too dark: could be blood in the bowel movement.

Quantity
More than usual.
Less than usual.

Unusual objects in the motion
Worms.
Bits of bone.

Odour
Certain intestinal infections may cause a particularly strong odour.

---

2 Abortion or Miscarriage

Miscarriages are infrequent among bitches, but they do occur as the result of an infection, a hormonal imbalance, an accident or as one of the results of poor feeding.

The condition occurs when the foetus is expelled from the uterus before the end of the normal gestation period, which is sixty-three days.

Early symptoms
As the birth process begins, the pregnant bitch will show signs of discomfort and restlessness, which will be accompanied by some bleeding from the vulva. This bleeding is followed by a clear discharge from the vulva. Then the miscarriage takes place, usually quite rapidly and painlessly, since the embryos are soft and small.

EMERGENCY

In some instances, fortunately rare, severe haemorrhage occurs during the birth or immediately afterwards. *This is an emergency.*

First Aid

(i) Try to staunch the bleeding by applying an absorbent pad to the vagina.

(ii) Keep the animal calm and quiet.

(iii) Get professional help without delay.

3   Abscesses

Description

An abscess is a swelling, caused by a collection of pus under the dog's skin. This swelling is accompanied by localized pain and heat. Normally, the swelling grows larger and larger until 'pointing' occurs. When this happens, the abscess softens and finally bursts.

WARNING

Do not squeeze an abscess. Allow it to burst naturally. An abscess is formed by the body in order to wall off an infection. When you squeeze the abscess, you are breaking down the wall and forcing the infection back into the body.

Treatment

Encourage the abscess to point by:

(i) Bathing it in a hot saline solution.

(ii) Applying hot compresses directly over it until it bursts. When it does burst, wash away the pus with a solution of 2 teaspoons (10 ml) hydrogen peroxide, Dettol, Savlon or TCP, added to 1 pint (500 ml) warm water.

With abscesses which do not drain completely, bathe every two hours with warm salt water, to keep the abscess open and draining. (Use 1 teaspoon (5 ml) table salt to 1 pint (500 ml) warm water.)

Specific Abscesses

The 'specific abscess' is found on

1   roots of the upper teeth

2   infected anal glands

Symptoms of tooth-root abscess

If an abscess keeps recurring below the dog's eye, or along the line of the upper jaw, examine the dog's mouth. A decayed tooth may be causing the abscess.

Treatment for a decayed tooth

There is no first aid for this condition. Tooth-root abscesses require extraction of the tooth and antibiotic therapy. See a vet.

Symptoms of gland abscess

Anal gland abscesses will cause very painful red swellings under the anus, on one or both sides.

Treatment for anal gland abscesses

(i) Apply hot compresses to the area for ten minutes at a time, four times a day, until the swelling subsides.

(ii) If the compresses are not effective after forty-eight hours, it may be necessary to lance the abscess. If a veterinary surgeon is not available, the owner may lance the abscess himself.

Technique for lancing

(i) Boil a single-edge razor blade for twenty minutes.

(ii) Clean the skin around the abscess with a disinfecting solution of Cetavlon and alcohol (1 teaspoon (5 ml) of each to 1 pint (500 ml) water).

(iii) Have an assistant hold the dog's head tightly, or, tie the dog's mouth shut (see **Restraint**).

(iv) Make a half-inch incision over the softest, reddest point of the swelling.

(v) Allow the abscess to drain.

---

4 Acute Middle Ear Infection

Cause

Usually seen as the sequel to originally simple ear complaints which have not been treated.

Symptoms

Loss of balance. The dog may walk around with its head constantly on one side, or it may have difficulty in standing.

Treatment

This condition is an emergency. The infection can spread

rapidly to the brain, causing severe meningitis, encephalitis and death. Antibiotics must be administered as soon as possible.

---

5   Acute Otitis

Often occurs after an ear-mite infection.

Symptoms
Symptoms may be similar to those of ear mites, but with severe inflammation. This condition is caused by a bacterial infection and treatment must be given by a professional.

Home treatment
To relieve the acute itching and soreness, pour warm olive oil into the ear. To relieve discomfort, administer one 300 mg aspirin tablet per 20 lb (9·10 kg) *body weight*, up to 1500 mg, once a day. See **Tablets and Pills: Techniques of Administration.**

WARNING
If left untreated, this condition can develop into a middle ear infection.

---

6   Allergies

General

Definition
An allergy is a reaction by the body to a substance to which it is oversensitive.

Causes
These substances include animal hair, plant pollen, certain drugs, certain foods, detergents and, not infrequently, the saliva of fleas.

Reaction
The physical reaction may take the form of vomiting, diarrhoea, dribbling, running eyes, redness of the skin, itching, lumps on the skin, and swelling of the lips and eyelids.

Treatment

The best way of treating an allergy is, of course, to remove the cause. In situations where this is not possible, either because the allergic substance cannot be identified or because it is in the air – such as pollen – then it is necessary to treat the allergic dog with the appropriate drug.

Most allergies respond well to antihistamines and corticosteroids. But the treatment must be given by a vet.

Respiratory Tract: Allergic Asthma

This is not a common condition, but when it does occur it must be treated.

Symptoms

Usually occurs in summer months. Affected dogs become very short-winded, wheezy and chesty.

Treatment

Administer antihistamines and adrenaline. (Dosage: Vallergan 1 mg/lb/453 g, adrenaline two to three drops, orally.)

Respiratory Tract: Hay Fever

Hay fever, an allergy of the nose and throat (upper respiratory tract), sometimes occurs in dogs.

Symptoms

Sneezing, accompanied by running eyes and nose, during periods of high pollen count. (Dates vary with locale.)

Treatment

Antihistamines (dosage: Vallergan 1 mg/lb/453 g) and corticosteroids.

Skin: Allergic Dermatitis

This condition is quite common in dogs.

Cause

An allergy to certain foods, varying from dog to dog. Hypersensitivity to flea bites is the main cause, however.

Symptoms

The dog develops sore, weeping, itching red patches, which often appear along the spine. If left untreated, the condition will not improve on its own.

Treatment

The object of the treatment is to break the itch-scratch cycle.
(i)   Shampoo the dog twice a week with a selenium-based shampoo such as Selsun.
(ii)   Apply liberal amounts of soothing lotion, such as calamine lotion, to the affected area twice a day.
(iii)   If the allergic dermatitis is caused by fleas, then get rid of them. See **Fleas**.
(iv)   Try to help the dog break the itch-scratch cycle by bandaging the paws, or putting baby bootees on them.
(v)   Obtain antihistamines and corticosteroid injections from a vet.

Skin: Nettlerash or Hives

Symptoms

This is an allergic reaction quite common in dogs. The effect is very sudden. The eyelids and face may become swollen; and round, clearly defined, raised patches appear on the dog's body.

Treatment

(i)   If the animal is not in great discomfort, treatment may not be necessary. Most cases of nettlerash clear up of their own accord in six to eight hours.
(ii)   If the condition does not clear up, the vet will administer antihistamines and corticosteroids. This should give the animal quick relief.
(iii)   If the hives are caused by an internal allergy, you won't be able to treat the condition at home, unless you know the allergen. However, if they are caused by stinging nettles, if the condition persists after twenty-four hours, and if professional help is not available, obtain a simple antihistamine cream from a chemist and apply it to the affected areas. Also, administer Diphenhydramine tablets, dosage 1 mg/3 lb/1·5 kg *body weight*. For elderly dogs and puppies give 0·5 mg/lb/453 g.

---

7   Amputation

Amputation is the removal of one or more limbs, either surgically or traumatically.

Surgical amputation

Severe fractures, bone cancers, or very severe cases of arthritis sometimes make amputation necessary.

Many dog owners are naturally reluctant to allow this operation, even though the animal's life is at stake. Some owners would rather have their pets 'put down' than have them hobbling about on three legs. If this reluctance is analysed, it usually turns out that the objection is basically due to the cosmetic effect of amputation. Owners faced with this decision should know that animals learn fairly rapidly to compensate for a missing limb and are able to manage quite well on three legs. As for appearances, it is amazing how quickly even the most sensitive dog owners become accustomed to their pets' missing appendages.

Traumatic amputation

This occurs during accidents.
1 A *tourniquet* must be applied immediately. See **Tourniquet.**
2 Measures must be taken to prevent or minimize the effects of *shock*, while the dog is being transported to the vet. See **Shock.**
If possible, have someone telephone the vet so that he can have the necessary transfusions ready when the animal arrives.

---

8   Anaemia

A blood condition characterized by the reduction of the oxygen-carrying capacity of the blood. There are three main causes of anaemia:
1 Loss of blood.
2 Red cell destruction (due to infection).
3 Poor blood formation (eg iron deficiency).

Symptoms

The dog is lethargic, shows no enthusiasm. The pulse is rapid. The animal is unnaturally pale around the eyes, nose and gums. See **Pulse Taking.**

The symptoms and their degree vary with the situation. A dog suffering from a debilitating disease will develop this unnatural pallor gradually, while a dog suffering from a haemorrhaging gastric ulcer will suddenly become very pale around the mucous membranes (see **Shock**).

Treatment

All anaemic animals need professional treatment.

If chronic anaemia is suspected and professional help is not available, administer ferrous sulphate tablets (obtainable from chemists) until you can have your dog examined by a vet. (Dosage: 30 mg per day for small dogs. up to 90 mg per day for large dogs.) (See **Body Weight of Dogs, Tablets and Pills: Techniques of Administration**).

9 Analgesics

Analgesics are used to relieve pain. When administering these pain-killers, pay careful attention to dosages.

When to administer
When the dog is in obvious pain or extreme discomfort.

Dosages
(i)   One tablet of 8 mg codeine per 20 lb (9·10 kg) *body weight*, to a maximum of four tablets a day.
or
(ii)   One tablet of 500 mg Paracetamol per 20 lb (9·10 kg) *body weight* to a maximum of four tablets a day.
or
(iii)   One tablet of 300 mg aspirin per 20 lb (9·10 kg) *body weight*, to a maximum of five tablets a day. See **Tablets and Pills: Techniques of Administration.**

10 Anal Glands

The anal glands, the size of a hazelnut, are circular glands located inside the anus at 4 o'clock and 8 o'clock position.
When the anal gland does not empty itself normally, it must be emptied by manipulation.

Symptoms of overfull anal gland
1   The dog continually smells of faeces.
2   It continually rubs its bottom on the ground.

Technique for emptying glands
(i)   Hold the tail in your left hand.
(ii)   With the right hand, make a ring of your index finger and thumb. Squeeze the ring with a slow but firm action against the base of the anus.

(iii) Discharge comes as the glands are emptied. The anal gland should not be emptied more than once every two months, or permanent damage may occur.

Anal eczema
When acute eczemas in this area are being treated, the anal glands should be suspected of causing the eczema and, as part of the treatment, the anal gland should be emptied.

Emptying the anal gland is not difficult, but it would be most helpful if the dog owner were to watch a vet do it once.

---

11   Anal Tumours (Anal Adenoma)

The anal adenoma is a locally malignant *tumour*.

Symptoms
This condition is seen only in older, male dogs. It takes the form of one or more swellings around the ano-rectal area or on the tail. In advanced cases, these swellings may ulcerate and haemorrhage.

Treatment
Effective and lasting treatment must be by a professional. In advanced cases, surgery may be required; in less advanced cases, antibiotics and hormones will probably help.
    While this condition is not an emergency, it must not be neglected. All too often, the dog owner is not even aware that it exists until his dog begins bleeding, and what was originally a simple problem becomes a more serious one.
    If bleeding occurs, hold a pad over the bleeding area and get the dog to a vet.

---

12   Anthropomorphism

Next to sheer ignorance, anthropomorphism is probably the second-ranking cause of improper medical home treatment.
    Anthropomorphism in this context is the fallacy of attributing human behaviour and mentality to dogs. While it is perfectly normal to speak of an animal as being 'nearly human', actually believing it can lead to serious errors of judgment, which in turn can lead to incorrect medical treat-

ment. If we think of a dog as a human being, we cannot properly observe and evaluate the animal's behaviour. In many instances, this makes it impossible to reach a correct diagnosis.

Dogs have their own psychology, their own patterns of behaviour and their own set of reactions. If we are to treat dogs intelligently, we must begin by thinking of them as dogs, and not as four-legged people.

13   Antibiotics

An antibiotic is a drug which kills the germs that cause certain infections. They are most effective when administered during the early stage of the infection. (Antibiotics are not usually effective against virus infection.)

Ideally, if your dog develops an infectious disease, the particular strain of bacteria responsible should be identified and the specific antibiotic administered. Unfortunately, disease states are rarely ideal, so a broad-spectrum antibiotic is administered. If there is no response within twenty-four hours, another broad-spectrum antibiotic is used, and possibly another, until a satisfactory response occurs.

14   Appetite

Increase in Appetite
A dramatic increase in appetite suggests

1   Simple greed, which may be due to a neurotic condition or, in certain cases, brain damage
2   Abdominal tumours
3   Diseases which prevent the food from being absorbed
4   Spayed bitches and castrated dogs tend to deposit more fat. These desexed animals need less food.

Treatment
Depends entirely on the cause. In the case of desexed dogs, feed them less than they want.

Loss of Appetite
It is not unusual for a dog to go off its food for twenty-four hours. But if the dog refuses food after twenty-four hours, remember, loss of appetite is a symptom of something else.

Check for:

1 Generalized disease
2 Tartar on the teeth
3 Foreign body in the mouth or throat
4 Sore mouth or sore throat. Look for sores in the mouth and red gums. Feel the animal's larynx. If it is sore, the dog will cough.

Treatment

Put the dog in a good light, or use an electric torch to examine the mouth and throat for obstructions. If there are no obstructions, then take the dog's temperature. If the temperature is elevated, a vet should be consulted. If a vet is not available, try to tempt the dog's appetite with succulent tasty treats like boiled boned chicken, strong cheeses, kippers, essence of beef (Brands Essence).

15   Artificial Respiration

Artificial respiration does the work of normal breathing: shifting air into and out of the animal's lungs. It should be administered as soon as it is observed that the animal is not breathing. Delay can be fatal. Within two to three minutes after breathing stops, the animal will be beyond recovery.

Technique

(i)   Lay the animal on its right side.
(ii)   Open the animal's mouth and check to be sure that there are no obstructions to breathing. If there are obstructions (sand, gravel, etc) pull them out with your finger. Make sure that the tongue is lolling out, clear of the back of the throat.
(iii)   Place the flat of both hands below the shoulder blade and over the ribs.
(iv)   Press down firmly, to empty the lungs.
(v)   Release the pressure. The lungs should fill as the natural elasticity of the chest returns it to its normal position.
(vi)   Repeat pressing down and releasing the pressure every five seconds until the dog is breathing on its own again. This could take up to an hour.
(vii)   The movements should be brisk and forceful. Press down hard. Release suddenly.

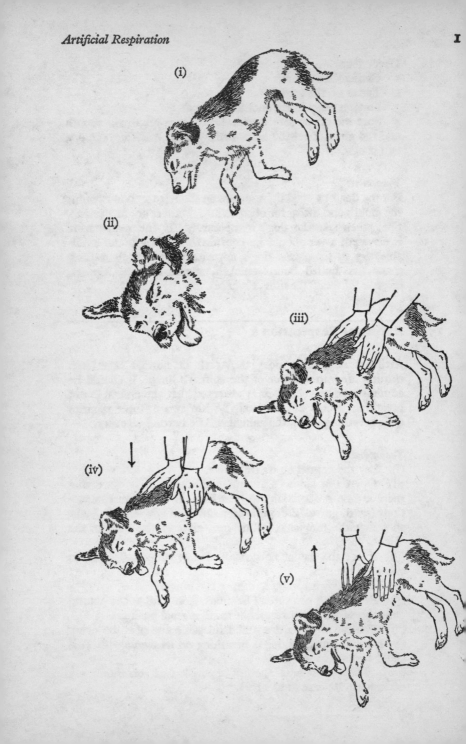

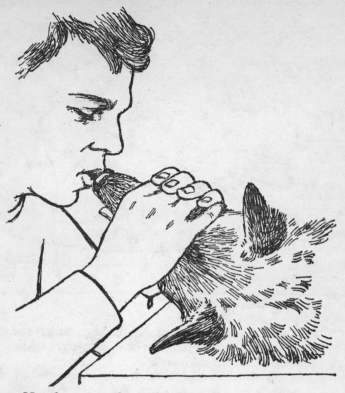

Mouth-to-mouth respiration

It is simple enough. Just hold the dog's mouth closed and blow into its nostrils. Wait a second, and blow again.

The idea is to inflate the animal's lungs with air so that they function of their own accord.

Swinging technique

With pups and small dogs, the technique is:

(i)   Slap the dog sharply on the side once or twice.

(ii)   Then lift the dog by its hind legs, extend your arms and swing it back and forth ten times (see illustration). Wait a few seconds for a gasp. If there is none, swing the animal again.

(iii)   When you swing a dog in this way, the weight of the abdominal contents will contract and expand the lungs. If, after four such swinging sessions, the dog is still not breathing, then administer mouth-to-mouth respiration.

16   Bad Breath (Halitosis)

As a general rule, an animal with bad breath is not well. If the condition persists for more than forty-eight hours, professional advice should be sought.

In animals under six months of age, bad breath sometimes accompanies the teething stage. But it also may indicate a worm infestation. With older animals, bad breath may indicate a number of disease states: tonsillitis, stomach infection, stomatitis (an ulcer of the mouth), infected or broken teeth, labial eczema (a condition of the lips, fairly common in spaniels), or sinusitis.

With elderly dogs, continuing halitosis may indicate a degree of chronic kidney failure.

Treatment
First, so far as possible, check for disease states. Does the animal 'act' sick? Is it feverish? Apathetic? Once these disease states have been eliminated as possible causes for bad breath, treat the condition by administering chlorophyll tablets or charcoal tablets. Dosage: one to six tablets a day, depending upon size (one tablet per 10 lb (4·5 kg) *body weight*, up to six tablets per day).

17   **Baldness (Alopecia)**

Causes
This condition is not uncommon in dogs and may occur without any visible cause. Baldness may be the result of an iodine deficiency, a hormonal imbalance or certain generalized illnesses.

Symptoms
The hair begins to fall out in patches. These patches may or may not itch.

Treatment
(i)   Apply a solution of 1 teaspoon iodine crystals mixed with 1 pint (500 ml) glycerine until dissolved.
(ii)   The vet may administer an oral dosage of thyroid hormone: 30 mg per 10 lb (4·5 kg) *body weight*.
(iii)   Oral administration of corticosteroids will also help to relieve the itching, but must be prescribed by a vet.

18   **Bandaging**

Bandages are used to
1   Stop bleeding.
2   Support injured legs.
3   Prevent the animal biting at its injuries.
4   Reduce swelling.
5   Prevent bacteria from entering a wound and causing infection.

Preferred type of bandage
The easiest type of bandage to use is the roller bandage, available in 12 and 15 ft (4 and 5 m) lengths, and in a variety of widths.

For bandaging dogs, the most useful width is the 2 or 3 in (5 or 7·5 cm) roller bandage.

For wounds on the trunk of the dog, the 5 in (12 cm) bandage is suggested.

It is sensible to keep a few different types of bandage in a handy first aid kit, but in emergencies, *any* wad of material will do.

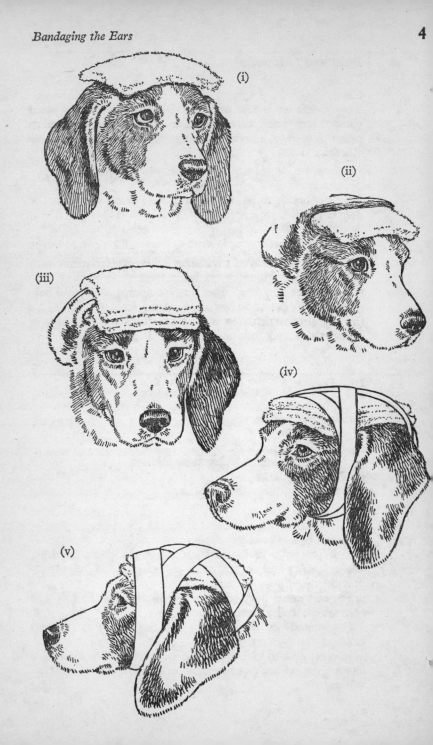

(i)

(ii)

(iii)

(iv)

(v)

Bandaging the Ears

Ears are rather difficult to bandage, but dog owners often have ample opportunity to practise, since a dog's ears are frequently torn after fights with other dogs and tend to bleed profusely, especially when the injured animal shakes its head.

Technique

(i)   Place a pad of cotton wool on top of the dog's head.

(ii)   Fold the affected ear over the pad.

(iii)   Place another pad of cotton wool over the ear.

(iv)   Wind the bandage around the head several times, leaving the unaffected ear in its normal position.

(v)   Anchor the bandage with a strip of 2 or 3 in (5 or 7·5 cm) elastoplast, placed on the top of the head.

(vi)   Care must be taken to ensure that the bandage is not wound too tightly, and does not affect the animal's breathing.

Bandaging the Eye

Technique

(i)   Place a moist gauze pad over the affected eye.

(ii)   Wind the bandage around the dog's head, leaving the ears in their normal position.

(iii)   Extend the bandage forward to cover the gauze dressing over the affected eye.

(iv)   Anchor the bandage with a strip of 2 or 3 in (5 or 7·5 cm) elastoplast, placed at the top of the dog's head.

(v)   Take care not to wind the bandage too tightly and be sure that it does not interfere with the dog's breathing.

Bandaging the Leg

Technique

When bandaging the leg, you should bandage the foot as well, in order to prevent swelling and tissue damage.

(i)   Pack the spaces between the dog's toes with small wads of cotton wool to prevent damage to the toes.

(ii)   Wrap cotton wool around the foot.

(iii)   Begin bandaging at the top of the leg, go down the front of the leg, around the foot and up the back (see illustration). Then wind the bandage around the leg, each layer of bandage overlapping the preceding layer, until the whole leg is covered.

(iv)   Tie off the bandage.

(v)   The bandage should be wound firmly enough not to slip, but not so tightly that it stops the circulation, unless it is a

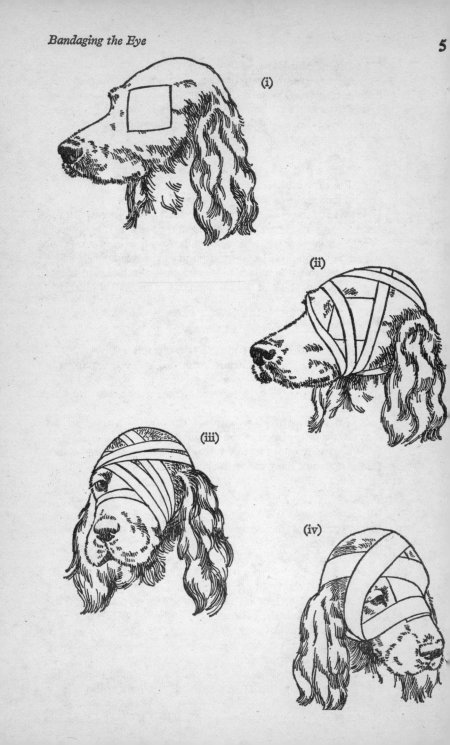

(i)

(ii)

(iii)

(iv)

(i)

(ii)

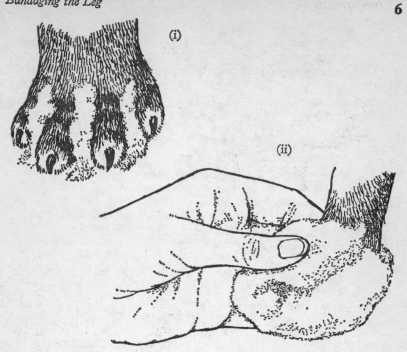

(iii)

(iv)

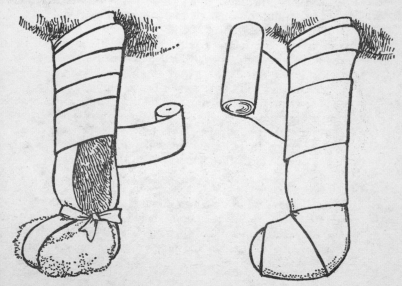

pressure bandage intended to stop a haemorrhage, in which case it should be checked every thirty minutes until the bleeding stops. Do not unwind the bandage completely, or you may reopen the wound.

---

19   Birth

Generally, birth occurs sixty-three days after conception, though on occasion a bitch may give birth a week early or a week late.

Signs of approaching birth
1 Approximately six hours before birth, the mother becomes restless and begins bedmaking. Bedmaking means preparing a place to give birth in (usually the most inconvenient place).
2 Vomiting may occur.
3 The animal's body temperature drops three degrees to about 98°F (36°C).
4 The vulva becomes enlarged and pinkish.
5 The pelvic ligaments slacken, causing some loss of co-ordination of the hind legs.

Various stages of labour
1 Within an hour before birth, the mother grows increasingly nervous, and may start glancing at her flanks. There are occasional contractions of the abdomen – one contraction every ten minutes, becoming more frequent.
2 The bitch lies down as the contractions become more frequent. As the foetus enters the pelvis, there is definite straining. The water bag, which looks like a black grape, appears at the vulva.
3 The mother will lick the water bag to rupture it. After the water breaks, the nose and feet of the puppy will appear protruding from the vulva.
4 After violent expulsive efforts by the mother, the infant dog is born. Often the mother will yelp or cry out as the puppy's head comes through.

Complications
(i) If there is more than two minutes' delay after the head and front legs are out, the puppy should be gently pulled out. Use a towel to grip without slipping. Grip as high as you can. It is essential to extract the puppy quickly and carefully.

(ii) Some puppies are born head first, some are born tail first. Both positions are normal, but if the puppy is born tail first, it should come out fairly rapidly. After the waters have broken, the puppy should be out within five to ten minutes. If it is not out in ten minutes, telephone a vet.

(iii) If the puppy is born with the membranes surrounding it still intact, and the mother does not remove them, remove them rapidly.

(iv) Every puppy should be checked before the mother has finished licking it, to be sure its mouth is free of mucus, enabling it to breathe freely.

(v) If breathing does not occur at once, rub the puppy briskly with a rough towel.

If this does not work, try mouth-to-mouth respiration.

Or place the puppy in a bowl of warm water and then plunge it into a bowl of cold water.

Do not give up for at least twenty minutes.

(vi) Once breathing has begun, put the puppy back with its mother and let her lick it dry.

(vii) She may try to eat the membranes, but you should

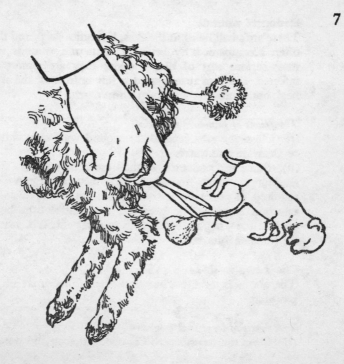

allow her to eat only one set (see **Mother Dog eating her Puppies**).

Umbilical cord
The umbilical cord should break when the puppy comes out of the membranes. If it does not break, tie it off with clean boiled cotton, 2 in (5 cm) from the puppy, and cut it off on the side of the knot farthest away from the puppy.

After birth
After the puppy is born, more membranes may be expelled. A greenish discharge, several hours after giving birth, is quite normal.

---

20 Bites, Fight Wounds

There are two types of wounds received from dog or cat bites:
Puncture wounds
Lacerated wounds

Puncture wounds
These are small holes in the skin, but quite deep, and they are often accompanied by bruising. Puncture wounds are the most serious sort of bite-wounds; they are almost always infected. If a puncture wound is left untreated, the skin will heal, but an abscess will form underneath.

Treatment of puncture wounds
(i) Clean the area around the wound with soap and water, or Cetavlon and water.
(ii) Since the puncture wounds are nearly always infected, antibiotics, which should be administered by a vet, are required. If professional assistance is not available, and if the infection seems to be growing, oral antibiotics should be given. Give 5 mg/2½ lb/1 kg *body weight* penicillin, twice a day for three or four days.

Lacerated wounds
The wound is jagged. The skin is torn. There may be profuse bleeding.

Treatment of lacerated wounds
(i) Clean the wound with Cetavlon, or soap and water.

(ii)   Check to be sure that the wound has drained and that there is no infection left. If the wound is discharging pus, it is still infected.

(iii)   If the wound is very large, it may require stitches.

21   Bitten Tongue

A bitten tongue is frequently seen in a dog and can be very serious.

Symptoms
Profuse bleeding from the mouth.

Treatment
A bitten tongue may sound like a minor mishap, but if the bleeding is very heavy, then it must be considered an emergency. Since the tongue is constantly moist and moving, it is difficult for a blood clot to form, so the bleeding is continuous; and if the cut is deep enough, the dog may bleed to death. Fortunately, it would take several hours, at the least, for this to happen, which gives you plenty of time to get the dog to a vet.

   If it is possible, that is, if the dog will allow it, hold its tongue in a cotton pad to reduce the bleeding, while you are transporting the animal to the vet.

22   Bladder Infection (Cystitis)

Fairly common in dogs.

Symptoms
1   Blood or traces of blood in the urine.
2   Passing urine with increased frequency.
3   Straining to pass urine.
4   Loss of appetite.
5   Abdominal pain.
6   In later stages, the urine will be heavily stained with blood.
As the disease progresses, pure blood will be passed.

Treatment
Do not feed the dog until professional help is available. In the event that it takes longer than twenty-four hours to get to a

vet, glucose and water may be given. Mix 3-4 tablespoons glucose powder with 1 pint (500 ml) water, and give one or two tablespoons (25 or 50 ml) of this mixture every two hours. See **Urethral Obstructions; Bladder Stones (Cystic Calculi)**

23   Blindness

Sudden blindness is a result of either a stroke or an accident in which the brain or the eyes themselves have been injured.

Temporary blindness occurs during infections of the clear part of the eye, ie keratitis. These infections, if not properly treated, can give rise to milkiness and eventually to ulceration of the cornea. If this (corneal) ulcer occurs, immediate professional treatment is vital. Do not bathe the eye: this might cause the ulcer to rupture.

Corneal ulcers take a long time to heal, and the dog may be left with a black scar on the cornea. The condition frequently occurs in breeds with bulbous eyes, such as Pekes and Pugs.

Progressive blindness is more common. It is usually the result of old age causing the formation of cataracts. However, these cataracts could also be caused by diabetes mellitus. See **Diabetes.**

Treatment
If you suspect that your dog is going blind and, of course, the symptoms are painfully obvious – bumping into things, unable to recognize people at a distance, etc – the first thing to do is to have the animal examined by a vet. He will be able to give you a definite diagnosis and, in case of cataracts, possibly improve the condition by surgery or enzyme injection.

But if the condition is irreversible, the dog owner should be aware that *blindness need not mean the end of the animal's life*. When the eyes fail, the other senses develop to compensate. Blind animals, as a rule, hear and smell much better than sighted animals. By the time the dog is completely blind, it will know its way around the house, and be able to go for walks, on the lead, of course. Blind animals, on the whole, manage remarkably well. They need just a little extra care. Most dogs, even those with normal eyesight, do not really see very well. In addition, dogs are largely colour-blind.

24   Blood Blister on the Ear (Haematoma)

Description

A thick, fluctuating, irregular swelling usually found on the inside of the ear flap, but the outside of the ear flap may be involved as well. The blister itself is painless and rather firmer than an abscess.

These blisters come up quite suddenly, usually as the result of a blow, a bite or as the sequel to an ear-mite infestation, or from an irritation which causes constant scratching. Such an irritation might be caused by an infection in the ear, in which case it will be accompanied by pus coming from the ear canal.

Treatment

(i)   If the blister is the result of an ear infection and is small, then leave it alone and treat the infection (see Index for ear infection).

(ii)   If the blood blister is not the result of an infection and is small, then just bandage it. Quite often the bandaging will cause the blister to be absorbed naturally.

Technique
See **Bandaging the Ear.**

Treatment for persistent blister

(i)   If the blister has not disappeared after being bandaged for three or four days, minor surgery will be required to drain, curette and suture it.

(ii)   If the persistent blister is fairly small (about 1 in (2·5 cm) in diameter), you can drain it yourself:

(a)   Sterilize a needle by boiling it for twenty minutes.

(b)   Wash your hands.

(c)   Prick the blister on the inside of the ear flap with the sterile needle and allow it to drain naturally. Do not squeeze it.

(iii)   After the blister drains, bandage the ear to prevent infection and further irritation.

(iv)   With larger blisters (more than 1 in (2·5 cm) in diameter), it is advisable to seek professional assistance.

Blood blisters (haematomas), while not serious in themselves, can easily cause permanent disfigurement of the ear. The best first aid is to keep them bandaged and taped to the dog's head to prevent the animal from worrying them and making them worse than they already are. If the dog absolutely insists upon worrying them, use an Elizabethan collar.

25   Blood in Bowel Movement

A small amount of blood in faeces is seen from time to time in all meat-eating animals. Larger amounts of blood in the motion, however, are not normal and should not be ignored.

Causes
Blood in the faeces may be the result of an anal impaction, due to bones, or it may be caused by tumours of the rectum, canine virus hepatitis, poisoning or accidents.

Symptoms
If the blood found in the motion is bright red and fresh, it comes from the anal region.
   If the blood is black, it comes from the intestines.

Treatment
Unless the cause can be easily identified and treated, such as bones or a simple cut, have a vet examine the dog.
   Give no food until the bleeding stops.

26   Blood in Vomit

Causes
Fresh blood in vomit may be caused by accidents, tumours, or by foreign bodies which have cut the mouth, throat or gullet.
   If the blood found in the vomit is black, then it comes from the stomach or from the small intestine, and may be caused by a stomach ulcer or by tumours.

Treatment
There is no home treatment for this condition since it is not possible for the dog owner to accurately diagnose the cause.
   As a temporary measure, the dog should not be fed until a vet has examined it. If the vet cannot be seen within twenty-four hours, withhold food and put the dog on a glucose and water ration. Mix 4 oz (113 g) glucose with 1 pint (500 ml) water. Small dogs should be given 4 oz (100 ml), large dogs 1 pint (500 ml) of the mixture. Give once only in a twenty-four hour period.

27   Body Weight of Dogs

Hound Group

Afghan hounds	60+ lb (27+ kg)
Basenjis	21–25 lb (9·5–11·26 kg)
Basset hounds	40–50 lb (18–22·5 kg)
Beagles	40 lb (18 kg)
Bloodhounds	80–90 lb (36·24–40·77 kg)
Borzois	60+ lb (27+ kg)
Dachshunds (standard)	25 lb (11·26 kg)
Dachshunds (miniature)	11 lb (4·98 kg)
Deerhounds	85–105 lb (38·5–47·79 kg)
Elkhounds	50 lb (22·5 kg)
Finnish spitz	40 lb (18 kg)
Foxhounds	70 lb (31·71 kg)
Greyhounds	60–70 lb (27–31·71 kg)
Harriers	70 lb (31·71 kg)
Irish wolfhounds	120+ lb (54·35+ kg)
Otterhounds	65 lb (29·26 kg)
Rhodesian ridgebacks	85 lb (38·5 kg)
Salukis	50 lb (22·5 kg)
Whippets	20 lb (9·06 kg)

Terrier Group

Airedale terriers	50+ lb (22·5+ kg)
Australian terriers	10+ lb (4·5+ kg)
Bedlington terriers	18–23 lb (8·15–10·42 kg)
Border terriers	13–15½ lb (5·89–6·98 kg)
Bull terriers (miniature)	20 lb (9·06 kg)
Cairn terriers	14 lb (6·34 kg)
Dandie Dinmont terriers	18 lb (8·15 kg)
Fox terriers (smooth) Fox terriers (wire-haired) }	16–18 lb (7·25–8·15 kg)
Irish terriers	27 lb (12·23 kg)
Kerry Blue terriers	30–40 lb (13·5–18 kg)
Lakeland terriers	17 lb (7·70 kg)
Manchester terriers	20 lb (9·06 kg)
Norfolk terriers	15 lb (6·76 kg)
Norwich terriers	12 lb (5·43 kg)
Scottish terriers	19–23 lb (8·61–10·42 kg)
Sealyham terriers	18–20 lb (8·15–9·06 kg)
Skye terriers	24–30 lb (10·87–13·5 kg)
Staffordshire bull terriers	28–38 lb (12·68–17·21 kg)
Welsh terriers	20 lb (9·06 kg)

| West Highland White | 15–18 lb (6·76–8·15 kg) |

Toy Group

Chihuahuas (long coat) }	6 lb (2·72 kg)
Chihuahuas (smooth coat) }	
English toy terriers	8 lb (3·62 kg)
Griffons Bruxelles	6–9 lb (2·72–4·08 kg)
Italian greyhounds	6–8 lb (2·72–3·62 kg)
Japanese	4–9 lb (1·81–4·08 kg)
King Charles spaniels	10–18 lb (4·5–8·15 kg)
Maltese	5–7 lb (2·26–3·17 kg)
Miniature pinschers	10 lb (4·5 kg)
Papillon	3–7 lb (1·36–3·17 kg)
Pekinese	7–12 lb (3·17–5·43 kg)
Pomeranians	3–5 lb (1·36–2·26 kg)
Pugs	14–18 lb (6·34–8·15 kg)
Yorkshire terriers	up to 7 lb (up to 3·17 kg)

Gundog Group

English setters	60 lb (27 kg)
Gordon setters	65 lb (29·26 kg)
Irish setters (Red)	60 lb (27 kg)
Pointers	50–55 lb (22·5–24·76 kg)
German short-haired pointer	45–70 lb (20·26–31·71 kg)
Retrievers (Labrador)	70 lb (31·71 kg)
Spaniels (clumber)	55–70 lb (24·26–31·71 kg)
Spaniels (cocker)	25–28 lb (11·26–12·62 kg)
Spaniels (field)	35 lb (15·76 kg)
Spaniels (Irish water)	30–40 lb (13·5–18 kg)
Spaniels (springer, English)	40–50 lb (18–22·5 kg)
Spaniels (Sussex)	45 lb (20·26 kg)
Weimaraners	45–65 lb (20·26–29·26 kg)

Non-sporting Group

Alsatians (German shepherd)	up to 90 lb (up to 40·5 kg)
Bearded collies	up to 50 lb (up to 22·5 kg)
Boston terriers	15–25 lb (6·76–11·26 kg)
Boxers	60 lb (27 kg)
Bulldogs	50–55 lb (22·5–24·76 kg)
Bullmastiffs	110–130 lb (49·88–58·94 kg)
Chow-chows	60 lb (27 kg)
Collies (rough)	50 lb (22·5 kg)
Collies (smooth)	50 lb (22·5 kg)
Dalmatians	50–55 lb (22·5–24·76 kg)

Dobermans	60–100 lb (27–45·35 kg)
French bulldogs	28 lb (12·68 kg)
Great Danes	120+ lb (54·35+ kg)
Keeshonds	40 lb (18 kg)
Mastiffs	120+ lb (54·35+ kg)
Newfoundlands	150 lb (67·85 kg)
Poodles (standard)	50+ lb (22·5+ kg)
Poodles (miniature)	10 lb (4·5 kg)
Poodles (toy)	up to 10 lb (up to 4·5 kg)
Pyrenean mountain dogs	100–125 lb (45·35–54·35 kg)
St Bernards	120+ lb (54·35+ kg)
Samoyeds	45–55 lb (20·26–24·76 kg)
Shipperkes	12–16 lb (5·43–7·25 kg)
Schnauzers	30 lb (13·5 kg)
Miniature schnauzers	15 lb (6·76 kg)
Old English sheepdogs	80–100 lb (36·24–45·35 kg)
Shetland sheepdogs	10 lb (4·5 kg)
Shih Tzus	14–16 lb (6·34–7·25 kg)
Tibetan Absos	12–15 lb (5·43–6·76 kg)
Tibetan spaniels	9–16 lb (4·08–7·25 kg)
Tibetan terriers	14–30 lb (6·34–13·5 kg)
Welsh corgis (Pembroke)	20–24 lb (9·06–10·87 kg)
Welsh corgis (Cardigan)	22–26 lb (9·96–11·78 kg)

---

28 Breaking Wind (Flatulence)

This condition occurs with dogs which are:

1 Overweight
2 Underexercised
3 Suffering from a dietary imbalance
4 Suffering from a bowel infection

Treatment
(i) If your dog is older, and you have been feeding it one large meal a day, start feeding it two or three smaller meals per day. Check (see **Diet**) to be sure that you are not over-feeding.
(ii) More exercise (recommended for both dog and owner).
If reducing the size of meals and increasing exercise does not help, then:
(iii) Add a handful of charcoal to the dog's food each day.
(iv) Remove liver and heart from the diet.

EMERGENCY

Occasionally an animal will break wind excessively and will suddenly become quite bloated. Its abdomen becomes swollen with gas, and hard. *This is an emergency.* Death may follow from torsion (twisted stomach). Do not poke or probe the distended abdomen.

EMERGENCY TREATMENT

There is no effective first aid for this acute condition. The dog must be taken to a vet at once.

29 Breed Failings

A breed failing is an inherited physical defect and is due largely to indiscriminate mating of a faulty stock.

To some extent, hereditary diseases and failings are found in all breeds, but some are seen more frequently in certain breeds.

Hip dysplasia (an hereditary condition of the hip joint which causes lameness)
Alsatians, Samoyeds, Retrievers: Labrador and Golden

Patella luxation (dislocation of the knee-cap)
Cairns, Pekinese, Poodles, Yorkshire terriers

Entropion (turned-in eyelids)
Spaniels, Chow-chows, Retrievers, Boxers, Poodles

Progressive retinal atrophy (PRA) – (an hereditary condition of the eyes, leading to blindness)
Poodles, Retrievers, Spaniels

Prolonged soft palate (causes rattling in the throat)
Bulldogs, Pugs, Pekinese, Boxers

Labial eczema (eczema of the lips)
King Charles spaniels, Red setters (Irish setters)

Luxation of the eye lens (lens slipping out of place)
Wire-haired fox terriers, Staffordshire bull terriers

30   Broken Back (Fractured Spine)

Fractures and dislocations of the spinal column almost never occur spontaneously. They are usually the result of some traumatic incident such as a car accident, a fall, or a blow with a stick across the back.

Symptoms
1   The dog will be unable to move its rear limbs.
2   It will be insensitive to pain below the affected portion of the spine.
3   There will be urinary and faecal incontinence and retention.
4   As a general rule, if the animal cannot move both back legs, if there is no response when the toe is firmly pinched, and if it has been involved in an accident, it is a fair assumption that the dog has a break or fracture of the spine.
5   The animal's front legs are usually extended.
These symptoms could indicate a slipped disc, but the slipped disc occurs spontaneously and not as the result of a traumatic accident.

Treatment
(i)   If the dog has been hit by a car, *do not move it unless it is absolutely necessary.*
(ii)   Telephone a vet, the police or the RSPCA.
(iii)   If you are unable to do any of these things, use the back seat of a car, or get a board large enough to place the injured animal on and then very gently *slide* the dog on to it. *Do not lift the dog.*
(iv)   Tie the dog on to the board by wrapping a bandage around the dog and the board.
(v)   Now lift the board and place it across the back seat of a car or on the floor if there is room, and drive to the nearest vet.

Prognosis
The outlook for dogs which suffer fractures and dislocations of the spine is not very hopeful. In the majority of cases, the dog will have to be put down.

31   Broken Tail

Fractures of the tail occur after accidents and with over-enthusiastic dogs confined to small areas.

Fractures of the root of the tail

If the break has taken place at the root of the tail, the whole length of tail will hang straight down. Also there will be some pain and swelling at the site of the fracture.

Treatment

The dog owner should not attempt to treat root fractures. Professional assistance is necessary. If the animal is in pain, administer one aspirin tablet for small dogs, up to 4 for large dogs, once only. Then get the dog to a vet.

Fractures along the length of the tail

Fractures of this type are easily identified. The tail, up to the site of the fracture, can be moved by the dog while that portion of the tail beyond the fracture will hang limply.

Treatment

If there is a delay of more than twenty-four hours before the dog can be seen by a vet, an elastoplast dressing should be applied to support the length of the damaged tail. Tape the break, tight enough to provide support but not so tight that the circulation is cut off.

Fractures of the tip of the tail

Again, an elastoplast dressing, taped around the fracture; again, be careful not to tape it too tightly. Leave the dressing on until the fracture mends.

It usually takes about three weeks for a tail fracture to mend.

It is important that dogs with fractures or suspected fractures of the tail be examined by a vet. Quite often, nerve damage is caused, and that portion of the tail beyond the fracture may have to be surgically removed.

32　Broken Tooth

Occasionally a dog breaks its tooth by biting too hard on something harder than its tooth.

This is not an emergency. Of course, the broken tooth may have to be extracted eventually. But meanwhile, there is one consolation: a broken tooth does not hurt. However, very cold or very hard substances may damage the exposed part of the tooth.

Symptoms
1 Dribbling.
2 Slight bleeding from the mouth.
3 Bad breath.

33 Bronchitis, Excessive Coughing and Kennel Cough

Symptoms
Excessive coughing, often with phlegm.

Treatment
(i) First, get a good light and examine the dog's throat to make sure that the cough is not caused by a foreign body in the mouth or throat.
(ii) Then, treat the cough with codeine linctus, 1 teaspoon (5 ml) per 20 lb (9·10 kg) *body weight*, three times a day.
(iii) Diet: no food for twenty-four hours. Then a light diet of fish, rabbit or chicken. If, after forty-eight hours, your dog is still coughing excessively, find a vet.

Kennel cough is a dry cough, unaccompanied by phlegm. It is caused by a virus which does not respond to antibiotics. If untreated, the dog usually coughs for five or six weeks before the condition recedes. But though the cough goes, if the condition is not treated the dog may be left with impaired breathing. So *when coughing persists, get a vet*. If professional help is not available, home treatment is an obligation.

Treatment
Administer codeine tablets: 8 mg per 20 lb (9·10 kg) *body weight*, to a maximum of 40 mg per day, until the condition improves.

34 Bruises and Contusions

Description
Bruises and contusions are easy to see on the hairless parts of the animal, where the bruise appears bluish-red and is painful to the touch.

If the bruise is under the hair, you will not be able to see it, but you will be able to feel it and to judge just how severe it is by your dog's reaction.

Treatment

(i) Examine the area around the bruise for breaks in the skin; these cuts and abrasions are often seen in association with bruises. If you find any cuts, clean and dress them (see Index).

(ii) Apply hot compresses over the bruise for fifteen minutes, every two hours.

(iii) If the dog is suffering marked discomfort, administer an analgesic.

---

35 Burns and Scalds

Burns and scalds are the most common household accidents and the pet owner should familiarize himself with the treatment of these mishaps *before* they happen.

A burn is caused by dry heat, such as a flame. A scald is caused by moist heat, such as steam. But the difference is academic since the symptoms and the treatment are the same for each.

Treatment

(i) When handling or treating a dog that has been burnt, be careful. Burns are very painful and animals in pain resent being handled. A good tape muzzle or a competent assistant is essential (see **Restraint**).

(ii) In serious cases, where the dog has been badly burned, treat first for shock. Keep the dog warm and give it a mixture of glucose and water.

(iii) Relieve the pain by administering analgesics.

(iv) Then clean the area around the burn with a dilute solution of Cetavlon (1 teaspoon (5 ml) to 1 pint (500 ml) water) to remove any damaged tissues (burnt or charred skin).

(v) Apply tannic acid jelly (available at chemists) or a solution of cooled strong tea to the burnt area.

(vi) Bandage the area to prevent further fluid loss. It is this loss of fluid that creates serious problems in burn cases.

(vii) In very severe cases, wrap the dog in a blanket and get it to a vet.

Long-coated dogs

If a dog with a long coat is burnt or scalded, it usually takes two or three days before any signs appear. After two or three days, a sticky green crust forms on the skin. *Do not pull this crust off*. It will come away of its own accord, leaving a large, pinkish, weeping area. If it does not come away, bathe it off or soak it off. Then the area should be cleaned and dressed. Use a little cod-liver oil on a cotton wool pad for the dressing.

In very severe cases with associated shock, a vet will give stimulants and plasma to combat fluid loss. (See **Shock; Car Accidents: Transportation of Injured Dogs.**)

Chemical Burns
Causes
Caustic soda, sulphuric acid, hydrochloric acid (spirits of salt), diesel oil, etc. (A note on diesel oil: animals often come into contact with diesel oil when they go under a parked truck.)

Description
1 A chemical burn resembles a scald. The wound is moist and oozing.
2 The hair around the burn usually sloughs off.
3 If the animal has tried to drink the chemical, there will be ulcers around its muzzle and tongue.

Treatment
(i) Use soap and water to wash the chemical off the dog's hair and skin.
(ii) For acid burns, apply dilute bicarbonate of soda to the burnt area. For alkali burns apply vinegar and water.
(iii) Apply cortisone cream or Cetavlon to the burn.

---

36 Calcium

The main function of calcium in the diet is to aid the growth and formation of teeth and bones.

Proper amounts of calcium in the diet of puppies are essential. A lack of calcium in the diet will cause ricket-like changes which include swollen, tender joints, arched back, and stiff legs.

Acute calcium deficiency in the lactating dog will produce a condition called milk fever.

Milk is a natural source of calcium. But a dog suffering from a calcium deficiency needs a concentrated dose and should drink a solution made with calcium borogluconate powder (available from chemists). Add 4 tablespoons (100 ml) of this powder to 1 pint (500 ml) water.

The dog will probably refuse to drink this voluntarily, so the owner should be prepared to force-feed.

---

37   Canine Virus Hepatitis

A highly contagious virus infection (transmittable only to other dogs). Unlike distemper, this form of virus has a low mortality rate.

The disease exists in four well-defined forms (worst first):

Fatal fulminating form
This form causes sudden death, after a rapid collapse, which is preceded by blood-stained diarrhoea.

Acute form

Symptoms
1 The dog is 'poorly' for four to six hours.
2 The dog is depressed, lethargic.
3 The dog may have a high temperature.
4 The dog may vomit blood.
5 The dog will have blood-stained diarrhoea.
6 After about six hours, if not professionally treated, the dog will fall into a coma and die.
Get the dog to a vet before the coma stage and there is a chance that its life may be saved.

Subacute non-fatal form

Symptoms
1 The dog's temperature is around 105°F (40°C).
2 Rapid heartbeat.
3 Tonsillitis.
4 Blood-stained diarrhoea.
5 Yellowing of the eyes and gums (jaundice).

Prognosis
Occasionally death does occur, but if the animal survives the first forty-eight hours, it will not die.

Subclinical form
In this form, there are no definite symptoms. The dog is simply out of condition: lethargic with little appetite. A blood

test is the only way of making a definite diagnosis.

Treatment
(i)   Professional help must be sought. The dog owner can only treat the symptoms as they arise, and often they pass unnoticed.
(ii)   Administer Vitamin B complex tablets. Give two tablets once a day for small dogs, up to five tablets twice a day for large dogs, for two weeks. Also give Vitamin B-12 tablets. Dosage is two tablets twice a day for small dogs, up to ten tablets twice a day for large dogs, for two weeks. These vitamins are helpful as a supplement to professional medical treatment. See **Tablets and Pills: Techniques of Administration.**

---

38   Capped Elbow and Bedsores

A common condition with larger dogs: Alsatians, Great Danes, mastiffs and St Bernards.

Cause
Lying on hard floors. Because of the dog's great weight, its skin is damaged and a protective reaction, the capped elbow, occurs.

Symptoms
1   A fluctuating, fluid-filled swelling develops at the elbow.
2   The hair around the swelling falls out and a thickening of the skin takes place.
3   Open sores (ulceration) may occur.
4   In later stages, the swelling becomes hard and fibrous.

Treatment
During the early stages of the swelling, apply cold compresses to the swelling. A capped elbow is not an emergency but it should not be ignored. If you let it go on for too long, surgical drainage and dissection may be necessary.

Preventive measures
If you have a large dog, make sure that it has a soft bed to lie down on.

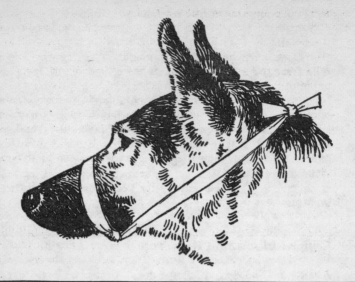

39 Car Accidents: Moving an Injured Dog

First consideration

Do not move the animal any more than you have to. Decide *where* you are going to move him to *before* you move him.

Moving an injured dog

Small dogs may be lifted by the scruff of the neck and carried. The best way to move a larger dog is on an improvised stretcher. The back seat of a car will serve. If there is no one to help you carry a stretcher, make a sling using your coat or a blanket and carry the animal in that.

Moving an animal in great pain is not the easiest thing to do, so be prepared for some problems. A badly hurt or frightened dog may bite anyone who tries to touch it, including its owner. Do not waste time trying to calm the dog with soothing talk: if it is really hurt, it will not hear you. Just take the proper precautions against being bitten and get on with the job.

Precautions

The best way to prevent a dog from biting you while giving it treatment is to tie its jaws shut. If the animal is hysterical, that is just what you will have to do. Use a short length of cord, a necktie or, if there is one, a bandage. Loop this around the muzzle and make a knot under the jaw. Carry the bandage back behind the dog's neck and tie the final knot just behind its ears. Now you can safely handle the dog (see **Restraint**).

Slide the animal on to the stretcher or into the sling and get it to the nearest vet. It is usually better and much faster to get the dog to the vet than to try to get the vet to the dog. If possible, have someone telephone the vet so that emergency treatment is ready when you arrive.

If you do not know a vet, call the police and they will tell you where the dog should be taken.

Warmth, no fluids

Try to keep the dog warm while you are getting it to the vet. Do not apply external heat; just keep the animal covered with a coat or a blanket. The idea is to prevent loss of body heat. Do not try to numb the pain by pouring whisky down the dog's throat, or try to counteract shock with warm milk or water.

Bleeding

If the dog is bleeding badly, try to stop or at least staunch the bleeding. If you can, determine whether the animal is bleeding from an artery or a vein. This is done by observing the way the blood flows.

Arterial wounds

If the blood comes out in a pumping fashion, in time with the heartbeat, and if it is bright red, then it is from an artery and the bleeding must be stopped or the dog will die.

For arteries, if the wound is on the limbs, make a *tourniquet* by wrapping a bandage, handkerchief or necktie round the limb, *above* the injury, and inserting a pencil or a screwdriver into the bandage. Then twist the tourniquet until the bleeding stops.

Venous wounds

Blood flowing from a vein flows regularly, as opposed to being pumped from an artery. It is dark red. If the blood is coming from a vein, the tourniquet is applied *below* the wound.

It is important to remember that a tourniquet should not be *too* tight, just tight enough to stop the bleeding. Loosen the tourniquet every ten minutes to allow the blood to get to the rest of the leg.

Bleeding, emergencies

Unfortunately, it is usually such a gory mess that you cannot always determine whether the blood is flowing or pumping. Often the wounds are on the body, where a tourniquet cannot be applied. So, unless the source of blood is obvious and can be easily tied off, the best thing you can do is the fastest thing you can do. Grab anything – bandages, a torn shirt, a handkerchief, even a package of tissues – and put it over the wound and hold it there with as much pressure as you can.

Internal bleeding

If the bleeding is internal, or the blood is flowing from its nose or anus, there is nothing you can do except keep the dog still and get it to a vet as fast as possible. (Try not to have another accident while you are rushing the dog to the vet.)

Further attempts at first aid will almost certainly do more harm than good. Broken or fractured bones need expert treatment. Leave that treatment to an expert. You concentrate on getting the injured dog to the expert.

NOTE

In Britain, if a dog is injured in a road accident, the police must be informed. By law, the dog's owner is legally responsible for any damage (a good point to remember next time you let your dog out on its own).

40   Cataracts

A cataract is an opacity and hardening of the lens of the eye, which prevents the light from passing through it.

Symptoms

1   A gradual, growing opacity or milkiness of the pupil.

Causes

1   The most common cause of cataracts is old age. Keep in mind that cataracts cause varying degrees of blindness. In an elderly dog, the lens may appear quite opaque and yet a certain amount of vision is still possible.

2   If cataracts appear in the eyes of younger dogs, a disease state such as diabetes must be considered.

Treatment

Cataracts, like every serious eye condition, must be treated by a professional. This treatment should begin as soon as the dog owner notices the cloudiness. Delay can prevent possible cure.

In many cases, a non-functional lens can be surgically removed, resulting in the return of a fair degree of vision.

If the cataracts are caused by diabetes, professional treatment of the disease may halt the growth of the cataracts. If old age is the cause, the vet may suggest waiting until the cataract 'ripens', and then operating on it.

---

41   Choking

Choking takes place when either the tongue or a foreign body blocks the back of the throat and prevents the dog from breathing. Choking often looks worse than it really is because the dog panics, which makes it choke even more, which makes it panic even more. . . . *Don't you panic too.*

Treatment

If the dog has passed out (from lack of oxygen) open its mouth and pull its tongue out. Make certain that nothing is blocking the windpipe. If there is some blockage, do not try to push whatever it is down the throat. Hook it out with your finger. Once the throat is clear, if the dog is still unconscious, artificial respiration should be given.

If the dog is conscious, hold it upside down, by its hind legs, and thump it on the back. This may dislodge whatever is at the back of its throat. If it does not, and the dog is still choking, open its mouth (see **Restraint**) and use your fingers to fish out the foreign object. If the object is stuck, pour a little olive oil down the animal's throat, to lubricate the gullet. If your probing causes the dog to gag, so much the better, as this may bring up the obstruction.

Prevention

Dogs often choke on those small, hard rubber balls that are given to them to play with. These are difficult to dislodge from the throat and should not be given. The softer, hollow type of ball is much safer.

Bones getting lodged sideways in the animal's throat are an even more common cause of choking. This can be prevented by not giving it bones. It is a common fallacy that bones are necessary for a dog's health. Quite the opposite. We do not recommend feeding bones.

42   Chorea or St Vitus' Dance

Seen as the sequel to distemper.

Symptoms
Pronounced and frequent twitching of a muscle or muscles, especially of the face and legs. Also, a clicking of the jaw.

Treatment
There is no known remedy for this condition.
    Fortunately, in mild cases, it does not trouble the dog, and it is not transmitted through breeding.

43   Clipping Nails

Technique
If the nail is black and the quick cannot be seen, cut along the line formed by the base of the nail (see illustration).

WARNING
Do not clip the nail too short or you will cut the vein under the nail and cause the toe to bleed.
    Should this happen, the bleeding can be controlled by bandaging the nail (see **Bandaging**) or by applying a silver nitrate pencil to the site of the bleeding.

44   Colds

Dogs do not catch colds. But if a dog exhibits the symptoms of the common cold, *do not treat these symptoms lightly*.
    The symptoms (runny nose, coughing, shivering, etc) suggest something more serious. (See **Distemper; Sinusitis**.)

45   Compresses, Cold and Hot

A compress is made by taking a wad of cotton wool or material

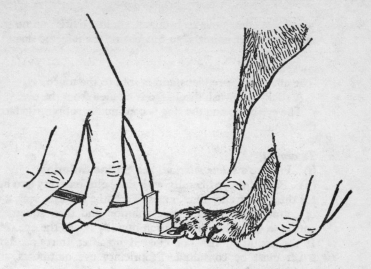

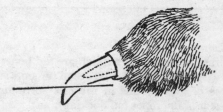

and saturating it in the proper solution.

Cold compresses or ice packs are applied directly over a swelling which was caused by a blow, and will bring the swelling down.

Hot compresses are especially effective for reducing pain. They are made by soaking cotton wool in the hottest water your hands can bear. Wring out the excess water and apply to the affected area for about two minutes. Repeat as often as possible.

Hot compresses relieve pain.

Cold compresses reduce swelling.

Hot and cold compresses can be used in conjunction with each other. For sprains and strains, use alternate hot and cold compresses.

46   Conjunctivitis

While not contagious to humans, conjunctivitis can be transmitted to other animals, so quarantine the infected dog.

Symptoms
The affected eye reddens and is sore to the touch.
    A sticky yellowish discharge is exuded from the eye.
    The eye hurts and the dog is continually rubbing its face on
the ground.

Treatment
(i)   Prepare a *saline solution*. See **Saline Solution.**
(ii)   Bathe the eye liberally with this solution every two hours
for the next twenty-four hours. To bathe the eye, soak a wad
of cotton wool in the saline solution and then squeeze the
cotton wool so that the solution literally floods the eye.
If the condition has not cleared up after thirty-six hours,
a vet must be consulted. Proprietary eye ointments, often
sold in pet shops, are not recommended.

47   Constipation

Causes
Often occurs in dogs which are fed bones; in male dogs with
enlarged prostate glands; rectal tumours; abdominal tumours;
loss of muscle tone in muscles surrounding the anus (as a
result of improper tail docking); anal gland abscesses; slipped
discs; and after badly healed fractures of the pelvis.

Symptoms
1   Straining.
2   Passing a brown, watery discharge.
3   Possibly bleeding from the anus.
4   Vomiting may occur.

Treatment
Administer 3–5 tablespoons (75–125 ml), depending upon size,
of liquid paraffin (an excellent laxative) and starve the dog.
    If the dog has not passed a motion within twenty-four
hours of receiving the laxative, contact the vet. The cause of
the constipation may be more serious and an enema may be
necessary.

48   Cough Medicine

A cough medicine is a product designed to soothe or suppress a cough.

Before administering cough medicines, take into consideration that a cough is not a separate entity, but a possible symptom of many diseases, and that treatment of the symptom will not remedy or remove the cause.

A cough medicine may stop the cough (temporarily) and allow the dog to rest. However, it will not cure whatever is causing the cough.

If possible, try to determine the cause of the cough before administering the cough medicine.

Possible causes of coughs
1   Tonsillitis.
2   Laryngitis.
3   Bronchitis.
4   Pneumonia.
5   Pleurisy.
6   Foreign body in the throat.
7   Distemper.
8   Chronic heart disease.

Dosage
2 tablespoons (50 ml) honey in 2 tablespoons (50 ml) water and 1 teaspoon (5 ml) lemon juice; or, codeine phosphate either as linctus (syrup) or in tablet form.
As linctus: 1 teaspoon (5 ml) per 20 lb (9·10 kg) *body weight*, three times a day.
As tablets: one 8 mg tablet per 20 lb (9·10 kg) *body weight* three times a day.

If, after forty-eight hours, the dog is still coughing, a vet should be consulted.

49   Cracked Pads

Symptoms
1   If a dog is suffering from a cracked pad, it will be lame on hard surfaces but sound when walking on grass.
2   Before you decide that your dog has a cracked pad, examine the paw carefully, in a good light, to be sure that it is not a *cut pad*. See **Wounds**.

Cut pads are much more common, especially in city dogs. Also check to be certain that the lameness is not caused by a cracked nail, particularly a dew-claw.

Treatment
(i)   Treat a cracked or sore pad by bathing the paw in a solution made of cooled strong tea (tannic acid) with 4 table-spoons (100 ml) witch-hazel added. Continue the bathing twice a day for one week.
(ii)   Rub a little olive oil into the pad. Then tie a baby bootee on to the paw for a few days. If the dog chews the bootee off, bandage the paw with an adhesive bandage (see **Bandaging**). If the dog worries the bandage, use an Elizabethan Collar (see **Elizabethan Collar**).
(iii)   It is helpful to walk the dog on grass if there is any around, rather than on hard surfaces, until the pad heals.
(iv)   As a general rule regarding a cut or cracked pad, if it is not bleeding, the less treatment the better.
(v)   After the cracked pad has healed, encourage the animal to walk. This will make the pad harden sooner.

---

50   Dandruff (Scurf)

Not uncommon in dogs with dry coats. Dog dandruff looks exactly like human dandruff; fine white flakes scattered through the coat, especially along the spine.

Treatment
This is a *skin condition* and should be promptly treated to prevent it from becoming a problem.

Shampoo the dog every three days for two weeks with a selenium-based shampoo (eg Selsun).

Also, give a small dog 1 tablespoon (25 ml) corn oil daily for a week; larger dogs, 2 tablespoons (50 ml) daily for a week.

Dogs with a tendency towards this dry flaking of their skin should have regular amounts of corn oil added to their diets: 4–6 tablespoons (100–150 ml) a week, depending upon size, should prevent the condition from recurring.

---

51   Deafness

Deafness, unfortunately, is fairly common in dogs.

Hereditary deafness
Usually seen in white animals, with blue eyes. Dogs suffering from hereditary deafness should be neutered to prevent them from passing on the condition.

Acquired deafness
Acquired deafness is often seen as the result of ear infections or accidents. It may be irreversible or temporary, depending upon the cause and the severity of the condition.

Partial deafness
Partial deafness is seen in elderly dogs and in younger ones which have ingested lead poisons.

Symptoms
Deaf animals may appear to be stupid. They do not respond to their names or to commands, and they are apt to bark continually.

A definite diagnosis of true deafness is difficult, since the deaf dog is compensated by the enhancement of its other sensory perceptions, especially the ability to detect vibrations.

---

52 Death

Eventually, all dogs die. The problem is how to be certain that the animal is dead.

Symptoms
1 Immediately after death, the dog's body is limp and flaccid.
2 The eyes are glazed, the pupils dilated. A light shone into the eyes gives back a green reflection.
3 There is complete absence of pulse, heartbeat and breathing.
4 Hold a mirror close to the animal's nose. If the animal is breathing, the mirror will mist over.
5 If the animal is dead, after a few hours its body stiffens, as *rigor mortis* sets in.
6 Eventually, decay begins.

53   Destruction

Animals in their natural, wild state rarely die of old age. Having extended the life-span of our dogs by protecting them as far as possible from illness and accident, we have the responsibility of caring for them in their old age, and finally of sparing them any unnecessary suffering.

A part of that responsibility is the decision as to when that point of unnecessary suffering has been reached. Chronic illness, incontinence, senility are the factors to be balanced against more subjective feelings such as the dog owner's love for his pet and the sanctity of life in general.

While the final decision is the individual owner's responsibility, too often people permit their old pets to linger on painfully, hoping that the poor old thing will die soon. When you find yourself feeling that way, perhaps it is time to do your old pet one last kindness.

When a dog is put down by a veterinary surgeon, the process is simple and painless. The dog is given an injection of an anaesthetic. Before you can count to three, the dog is dead.

The most difficult situations arise when a dog has been badly injured – usually in a car accident – and is in great pain. Most people are simply not equipped, mentally or physically, to destroy the animal. So, rather than take the chance of causing even greater pain, call the police at once. They will give you the emergency number of the nearest vet. Leave this sad job to him.

54   Dew-Claws

The dew-claw is a functionless toe that appears as a rudimentary claw placed on the lower, inside part of the dog's leg, just above the paw.

Since the dew-claws serve no purpose, and may catch on material, it is recommended that they be removed not earlier than three days after birth and not later than ten days. After ten days, professional assistance is required.

Technique for removing dew-claws in puppies
Puppies should have their dew-claws removed when they are three days old.
(i) Sterilize sharp scissors by boiling them in water for twenty minutes.

(ii)   Clean the skin around the dew-claws with a solution of dilute Cetavlon or alcohol.

(iii)   Then snip off the dew-claws.

Bleeding
If there is bleeding, sprinkle a few grains of potassium permanganate (available from chemists) over the area.

Removal of dew-claws in adult dogs
See a vet for surgery.

NOTE
Some show breeds require dew-claws, so owners of pedigree dogs should consult breed standards.

---

55   Diabetes

Cause
There is an abnormal amount of sugar in the blood, caused by a malfunctioning pancreas.

Symptoms
1   There is increased thirst and increased urination. A laboratory analysis would show traces of sugar in the urine.
2   There may be loss of weight.
3   There may be a sweetish odour of acetone (which smells like nail-polish remover) on the animal's breath.
4   There is an increase in appetite.
5   Secondary symptoms of cataracts may appear in the eyes.
6   If untreated, the animal may fall into a diabetic coma (see **Unconsciousness**).
A definite diagnosis must be made by a vet, after analysis of a *urine sample*. See **Taking Samples of Faeces and Urine.**

Treatment
(i)   Home treatment, after professional consultation, usually consists of daily injections of insulin (see **Injections**).
(ii)   Insulin should always be given *before* feeding.

Overdose
If an accidental overdose of insulin is administered, insulin coma will follow. This condition can be reversed by giving glucose or sugar by mouth. See **Force-Feeding.**

Drinking diabetes (Diabetes insipidus)
Cause
A disease of the pituitary gland.

Symptoms
1 The dog drinks vast amounts of water. *Be sure to keep its water bowl full.*
2 There is no smell of acetone on the breath.
3 The animal urinates frequently. The urine is very pale: laboratory tests will show that there is no sugar in the urine.

Treatment
The vet may put the dog on a course of hormone treatment.

See also **Kidney Failure.**

---

56   Diarrhoea

Dogs are natural scavengers and often suffer mild attacks of diarrhoea as a result of eating decayed foodstuffs, etc. However, diarrhoea can also be caused by viruses, bacteria or poisons.

Symptoms
1 Frequent passing of loose motions.
2 Foul-smelling motions.
3 The diarrhoea may be associated with vomiting.

Treatment
(i)   All foods and water should be withheld for twenty-four hours.
(ii) After twenty-four hours, give a cupful of water per day and small amounts of boned chicken and rice or fish and rice to eat for the next two to three days.
(iii) No milk should be given for one week.
(iv) If the diarrhoea persists, starve the dog again for another twenty-four hours. Then give the following mixture: Mix 3–4 tablespoons glucose powder, 1 raw egg white, 1 pinch salt into 1 pint (500 ml) warm water. Give the dog 2 tablespoons (50 ml) of this mixture every two hours for two days.
(v)   Put the animal on a reduced diet of chicken and rice, or fish and rice, for the next two to three days. Then resume normal feeding.

(vi)   Severe diarrhoea can also be controlled by administering tablets of codeine phosphate (obtainable from chemists): 8 mg per 20 lb (9·10 kg) *body weight*, three times a day.

Persistent diarrhoea

If diarrhoea persists for more than forty-eight hours, it may be the symptom of a more serious disease such as distemper or leptospirosis. A vet must be consulted.

Sore anus

Animals with diarrhoea may develop a sore anus. Cold cream or vaseline will help soothe the irritated area.

---

57   Diet

To maintain good health, dogs require a diet that includes carbohydrates, fats, proteins, minerals and vitamins in the proper proportions.

The simplest adequate ration is raw meat containing about 5 per cent fat, plus an equal amount of cereal in the form of biscuit meal.

Cooked, boned fish can be substituted for meat. Flaked maize or oatmeal can be used as an alternative to biscuit meal.

Canned foods mixed with an equal amount of cereal may be used in place of raw meat. These tinned foods are more expensive but more convenient. If tinned foods are used, do supplement them occasionally with a piece of fresh meat, particularly liver, to ensure proper vitamin intake.

An adequate tinned dog food will contain:
13 per cent protein
5 per cent fat
16 per cent carbohydrate
2·5 per cent ash

Feeding amounts

SIZE OF DOG	BODY WEIGHT		FOOD INTAKE	
	lb	kg	lb	kg
Small	10	4·5	$\frac{1}{2}$	0·25
Medium	25	11·25	$1\frac{1}{4}$	0·5
Large	40	18	$1\frac{3}{4}$	0·75
Very large	100	45	$2\frac{1}{2}$	1·1

This guide to feeding amounts is based on a mixed diet made up of 50 per cent meat (or meat substitutes) and 50 per cent meal or cereal.

Further, this guide is based on the assumption that the dog is getting enough exercise. If, for some reason, this is not the case, then the food supply should be reduced proportionately, up to half the normal amount for sedentary or elderly dogs.

Diet for Brood Bitch

A brood bitch is a bitch used for breeding.

Brood bitches may be fed their usual diet with extra milk and fat added. An extra pint (500 ml) of milk per day, plus two egg yolks, should be adequate.

Give one to two tablespoons of bone flour daily.

Do not feed the bitch biscuits from the day of mating until birth occurs. Biscuits, which contain carbohydrates, tend to make dogs fatter and a pregnant bitch should not be overweight.

Feeding Times

Dogs should be fed regularly at the same hour each day. In this respect they are creatures of habit, and at the accustomed hour their gastric juices begin to flow.

Puppies

Puppies should receive several meals a day.

At 8 weeks	4 meals a day
14 weeks	3 meals a day
18 weeks	2 meals a day
6 months	1 meal a day

Adult dogs

Grown dogs may be fed once or twice a day, depending upon the dog's appetite and upon the amount of exercise. Elderly dogs should be fed two or even three smaller meals, rather than one large one.

---

58 Discharge from the Penis (Balantis)

Cause

This condition is a result of an inflammation of the penis.

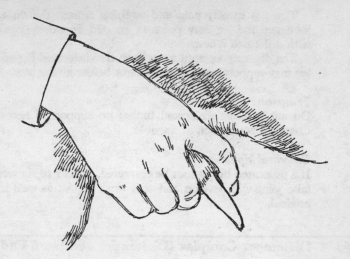

Symptoms
There is a continuing discharge or dripping of yellowish pus from the dog's penis.

Treatment
(i)   Pull the penis out of its sheath (see illustration) and bathe the head and exposed shank in a solution of dilute hexachlorophene, eg Phisohex, three times a day, until the inflammation and discharge disappear.
(ii)   If the animal will not allow you to pull out its penis, then syringe the inside of the sheath with a solution of 4 parts of water to 1 part TCP.
This syringing should be done three or four times a day until the condition disappears.

---

59   Dislocations

Dislocations occur when a bone has become displaced (pulled) away from the joint. They should not be confused with a *fracture*, which is a broken bone; and unlike fractures, most dislocations should not be splinted.

Symptoms
While a fractured limb tends to swing freely, the dislocated limb is more rigid.

There is usually pain and swelling around the dislocated joint and the leg may point in an odd direction, especially with dislocated elbows.

The dog may attempt to walk on the dislocated leg and the leg may support some of the weight before giving way.

Treatment
Do not bandage dislocated limbs; no support is necessary. Contact a vet as soon as possible.

Dislocated hip joint
If a dislocated hip cannot be corrected, in four to six weeks a false joint will develop and will work almost as well as the original.

---

60   Distemper Complex (Distemper and Hard Pad)

Description
Distemper is caused by a virus. It is highly contagious and any dog suspected of having distemper should be kept away from other animals.

Dogs of all ages are susceptible.

The incubation period is three to fifteen days.

Vaccination
The immunity produced by distemper vaccination lasts for about a year, so an annual injection is recommended.

Symptoms
1 Affected dogs become dull and apathetic.
2 The dog's temperature initially is very high, around 105°F (40°C).
3 No appetite.
4 There is a discharge from the eyes and nose. At first this discharge is watery. Later it becomes yellow and sticky.
5 The dog develops a dry cough.
6 At this stage the dog's temperature begins to fluctuate.
7 Conjunctivitis develops. (Conjunctivitis is an inflammation of the membranes around the eye.)
8 The nasal discharge dries into a hard greenish-yellow scab.
9 There is evidence of tonsillitis.
10 Vomiting.
11 Diarrhoea.

Second stage

Two to three weeks after the onset of the disease, the nervous symptoms appear:

1 These may take the form of convulsions, or of twitching of muscles on the dog's face and on the forelegs.
2 Circling may occur. The dog runs around and around. This stage may be associated with blindness and aimless wandering.

Treatment

Obviously professional help must be obtained.

The treatment depends entirely on the stage of the disease. The sooner the disease can be identified, the more hopeful the outcome.

The only treatment the owner can give is empirical, that is, to treat the symptoms as they arise.

Since distemper is a virus infection, antibiotics can only prevent secondary bacterial infections. The vet will also treat the disease with more specific and sophisticated drugs.

The success of any treatment for distemper depends largely upon the early identification of the disease. The later it is recognized, the less optimistic the prognosis.

Hard Pad

Hard pad is not really a separate entity. It is another example of how complex a virus infection can be.

Symptoms

Hard pad has the same symptoms as distemper, with the addition of:

1 Severe diarrhoea.
2 Hardening of the foot pads and the nose, occurring about fifteen days after the onset of the infection.

Treatment

Again, the success of the vet's treatment depends largely upon how quickly the dog owner realizes that his pet is ill.

---

61   Docking and Cropping

The cropping of dogs' ears is illegal in Britain, but in other parts of Europe and in the United States the docking and cropping of certain breeds is customary.

In the authors' opinion, this docking and cropping is nothing more than mutilation dictated by fashion. Further, docking a tail may cause chronic problems in the anal area.

However, if the owner insists upon docking or cropping, the operation should be performed by a qualified person.

---

62   Drowning

Treatment
Get the animal out of the water. Then:
(i)   If the dog is unconscious, lay it on its side and open its mouth; make sure that its tongue is out and that there is nothing obstructing the windpipe. Use your finger to check for grass, sand, mud, etc in the dog's mouth.
(ii) If the dog is still unconscious, lift it by its hind legs and allow the water to drain out of its mouth.
(iii) Administer *artificial respiration* or mouth-to-mouth resuscitation, which is slightly more effective. See **Artificial Respiration.**

---

63   Eczema

This common condition is a superficial inflammation of the skin and occurs in two main forms: acute and chronic.

Acute
Cause
Probably a severe allergic reaction.

Symptoms
1   Severe itching.
2   The hairs around the affected areas are broken and sparse.
3   The skin around the affected areas is bright red, moist and oozing. (In the long-haired breeds this may lead to the disease's going undetected, due to the matting of the animal's coat.)

Acute moist
Symptoms
1   Constant scratching.
2   This condition is typified by the sudden appearance of a large wet area exuding serum. (Serum is a yellowish fluid which dries to a yellowish crust.) Very painful breaks in the

skin can appear overnight. These lesions are most common in areas that the animal can scratch or lick, and they vary in size from a penny to a hand.

3 Initially, the breaks in the skin are wet and matted. Then they dry to a yellow scab.

4 The pain is acute and obvious. The dog is off its food and distressed.

Treatment

(i) Apply a solution of 1:1,000 potassium permanganate crystals to the area (a pinch of crystals to 1 pint (500 ml) water – available from chemists).

(ii) Wash the entire dog with a shampoo containing selenium, eg Selsun.

(iii) After drying the animal, dab calamine lotion on the affected areas.

Chronic

Causes

1 Dietary: excess carbohydrates; fat deficiency; vitamin deficiency.

2 Allergies.

3 In spayed females there may be scalding of the area around the vulva, by urine. This occurs because bitches spayed before their first heat often retain an infantile vulva which remains small instead of developing to adult size. (This, incidently, is one of the arguments in favour of not spaying bitches before they have had their first litter.)

4 Dirty skin.

5 Abrasions from collars or harnesses.

6 Friction between the elbow and chest.

7 Overwashing.

8 Hormonal imbalance.

9 Individual predisposition.

10 Breed susceptibility, eg as in Scotties and Jack Russells.

Symptoms

1 The affected skin becomes dry and flaky.

2 The affected skin is darker than the rest of the skin.

Treatment
Seek professional help.

Labial eczema
A form of eczema which attacks the lips and is particularly common in spaniels.

Symptoms
The lips become raw and red, with the surrounding hair on the muzzle becoming brown-stained and foul-smelling.

Treatment
(i)   Clip away hair around the lips.
(ii)   Wash the area well with soap and water daily. Any good-quality hand soap will do.
(iii)   For very severe cases: paint the sore areas with a silver nitrate stick (wear rubber gloves). If home treatment is not successful, surgery may be necessary to remove the folds around the lips.

---

64   Electric Shock

Usually caused by the dog's chewing on an electric cord. So, if you find your dog lying flat out next to a badly frayed electric cord, you will know to treat it for electric shock.

WARNING
Be careful! Very often a shocked dog urinates, and the pool of urine makes an excellent conductor. So do not step on it and do not touch the dog until you have turned off the current, or you will need someone to give *you* first aid.

If you are unable to turn off the electricity, put on a rubber glove or grab a thick dry towel and pull the electric plug out of the socket.

Or, if it is easier, get a wooden stick such as a broom handle and push the animal out of the urine and away from the electric cord.

Treatment
If the dog has not regained consciousness by this time, administer artificial respiration. Or, if the dog is small enough, try swinging first (see **Artificial Respiration**).

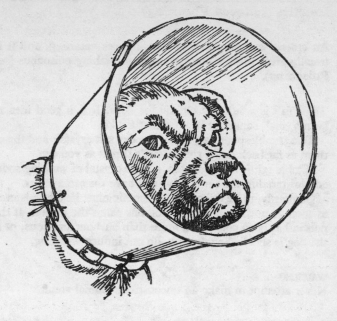

65   Elizabethan Collar

A most useful device when treating cuts, skin diseases, etc, an Elizabethan collar is used to prevent a dog from scratching at its face, ears or eyes, or to prevent it from biting various parts of its anatomy.

Classically, these collars are prepared from stiff cardboard; but this has obvious disadvantages, and we recommend plastic containers, varying in size from a small flowerpot for a small pup to a large plastic bucket for a large dog.

All that is necessary is to cut the bottom out of the flowerpot to a size that the head will go through. Punch four more holes around this hole, put strings through and tie the 'collar' to the dog's collar.

The open end must be sufficiently far away from the nose to prevent licking, and this may present difficulties when feeding time comes. If so, the collar can be removed briefly to allow eating and drinking.

The Elizabethan collar may sound and even look a bit horrific, but most dogs, after the first five or ten minutes, accept them quite calmly.

66   Emetics (Induced Vomiting)

An emetic is any substance that induces vomiting, and it is usually given after a dog has eaten something poisonous (see **Poisoning**).

Table salt is a suitable emetic for dogs. It is a good idea to keep a small container in your first aid kit.

Take 1 tablespoon (25 ml) of the dry salt crystals and throw them as far back down the animal's throat as you can.

If table salt is not available, a large crystal of washing soda, administered in the same way, will have the same effect.

Obviously, to be effective, the emetic must be administered as soon as possible after the dog has eaten the poison. If the poison has been consumed more than an hour previous, or if the dog is shocked or drowsy, do not induce vomiting.

WARNING
Never attempt to make an unconscious animal vomit.

67   Enema

An enema is an injection of non-irritant fluid into the large intestine, administered by way of the anal passage. The purpose of giving an enema is to empty the large intestine of any abnormal or impacted contents, so that the dog can pass a normal motion.

Enemas may be necessary after the consumption of a large amount of bones (not recommended feeding).

How to prepare an enema
The best enema solution is produced by lathering some good-quality soap into a dish of warm water (1 pint (500 ml) warm water with good-quality hand soap or soap flakes that contain no detergent).

The solution is administered into the anal passage by means of an enema pump.

If an enema pump is not available, you can improvise one, using a length of rubber tubing (approx $\frac{1}{3}$ in (1 cm) in diameter) leading to a plastic funnel filled with the enema fluid.

Technique

(i)   Spread some newspapers around the area *before* you give the enema; you will not have time afterwards.

(ii)   Have someone hold the dog. Enemas should only be given with the dog standing.

(iii)   Introduce about 3 in (8 cm) of tubing into the dog's rectum. A little vaseline on the end of the tubing helps.

(iv)   Hold the funnel higher than the dog.

Dosage

Administer up to 1 pint (500 ml), depending upon size of dog.

If substances that are causing impaction are not passed after three attempts, professional help should be sought.

---

68   Excessive Drinking (Drink-Vomit Cycle)

Symptoms

Increased thirst is a symptom of several conditions, all of them serious (see NOTE). Since the average dog owner is not competent to make a diagnosis, follow these general rules until a vet can examine the animal.

Treatment

Never withhold water from a dog with excessive thirst, *unless the dog is vomiting*. When a dog starts on the drink-vomit cycle, it will continue drinking and then vomiting until dehydration and death occur.

To break the cycle, withhold all water for twelve hours. Then give the dog 1 or 2 tablespoons (25 or 50 ml) – depending upon size – of a water and glucose mixture, every two hours for the next twelve hours. The mixture should consist of 3–4 tablespoons glucose powder dissolved in 1 pint (500 ml) water. (If glucose is not readily available, an ice cube may be given every hour.)

This treatment can be reinforced with codeine phosphate tablets: one 8 mg tablet per 20 lb (9·10 kg) *body weight*, twice a day, to a maximum of four tablets per day. If, after twelve hours, the dog is still vomiting, professional help must be sought.

NOTE

Other possible causes of greatly increased thirst are: diabetes; chronic interstitial nephritis; pyometra; increased body temperature; poisoning; enteritis; gastritis; other infections.

---

69   Eyeball out of Socket

This sometimes occurs after fights or road accidents, particularly in certain breeds with bulbous eyes (such as the pekinese, King Charles spaniel, bulldog, etc).

Treatment
(i)   Apply olive oil or vaseline to the eye socket and gently try to ease the eyeball back into place. Then bandage over.
(ii) If the eyeball will not fit, or will not stay in place, hold it in place with damp or oily cotton wool. (Saturate cotton wool with olive oil.)
(iii) Bandage over lightly. (See **Bandaging the Eye.**)
(iv) Get professional help.

---

70   False Pregnancy

This condition, to varying degrees, occurs in most bitches about nine weeks after the end of every heat period. It occurs because the ovaries of the female undergo the same changes as when mating and conception have taken place.

Symptoms
The symptoms of false pregnancy are exactly the same as those which occur during the final stages of a real pregnancy, with the exception of the abdominal enlargement (though this does occasionally occur). The mammary glands fill with milk. The bitch may try to make a bed or nest for herself. She may also start nursing woolly toys.

Treatment
(i)   Quiet her. Psychologically as well as physically, she is going through a difficult time. Administer half a 500 mg Paracetamol tablet for small dogs up to two tablets twice a day for large dogs.
  See **Tablets and Pills: Techniques of Administration.**
(ii) Add a pinch of Epsom salts to her food during this period. This will help her get rid of the milk produced by the false pregnancy. (It also might cause a mild touch of diarrhoea for a day or so.)

Severe cases

Severe or persistent cases will require hormone treatment from a vet. If the case is especially severe or recurs persistently, the owner should give the bitch contraceptive tablets to suppress the heat or have her neutered. Contraceptive tablets can be obtained from a veterinarian.

---

71 Feet

Dogs' feet are the equivalent of the soles of our shoes. But while leather soles wear out, dogs' feet do not. The pads are constantly growing and being resoled with dead, horny skin. Exceptions to this natural process occur after severe or prolonged exercise on a very rough terrain, or after an injury where the bottom of the pad has been sliced off.

If the bottom of the pad has been sliced off, allow it to heal naturally. Bathing will only soften the new skin that is forming and delay healing.

---

72 First Aid Kit

All dog owners should prepare a first aid kit and keep it in a tin, clearly marked and in a safe place. It should contain:
A pair of sharp-edged, blunt-pointed scissors
A pair of forceps (tweezers)
4 rolls of 2 in (5 cm) elastoplast
4 rolls of 2 in (5 cm) roller bandage
A packet of cotton wool
A packet of lint
A bottle of 20 vol hydrogen peroxide
A bottle of antiseptic, eg Savlon, Dettol, Roccal
A razor blade
A packet of needles
Codeine tablets
Paracetamol tablets
A packet of cotton buds
A crystal of washing soda (emetic)
Milk of magnesia
Table salt
An eyedropper
A copy of this book.

73 Fish-Hooks

If a dog gets a fish-hook caught in its mouth or anywhere on its body, take it to a vet at once if it is at all possible. It is easy enough to remove a fish-hook after the dog has had a general anaesthetic. Unfortunately, most fish-hook accidents happen in places remote from vets and it may be up to you to remove the hook.

Preparation procedure
(i)   Get someone to hold the dog. It is next to impossible to hold the animal and operate at the same time. So even if it takes a little longer, find someone to assist you.
(ii)   Get the best light you can. You must be able to see what you are doing.
(iii)   Get a pair of needle-nosed pincers or wire-cutters.
(iv)   Get a *sharp* knife or a razor blade. Boil it for twenty minutes.
(v)   Slip a tape muzzle over the animal's mouth and have your assistant hold the dog under the light (see **Restraint**).
   You are now ready to remove the hook.

Operative procedure
(i)   Look carefully at the way the hook is imbedded. Think about what you are doing before you do anything.
(ii)   *Do not try to pull the hook out.* If you do, you will tear a huge, bleeding chunk out of the dog.
(iii)   Determine which way the barb is pointing and push it out through the skin. Use the pincers or wire-clippers to snip off the barb of the hook. Then pull the hook out. Pull in the opposite direction from where the barb was pointing.
(iv)   If the hook is imbedded in such a way as to prevent you from getting at the head, you will have to use your sharp, sterile knife to make an incision over the area where the head of the hook is imbedded. Do not be too squeamish. Your incision will do a lot less damage than a forceful pull. After you have made the incision, use your pincers to snip off the head of the hook.
(v)   Dress the wound to prevent infection (see **Wounds**). This is unnecessary if the hook has been removed from the mouth or throat.

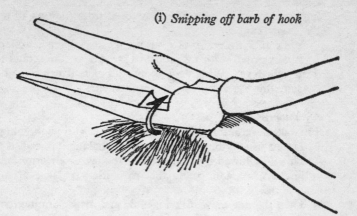

(i) *Snipping off barb of hook*

(ii) *Making incision before removing imbedded hook*

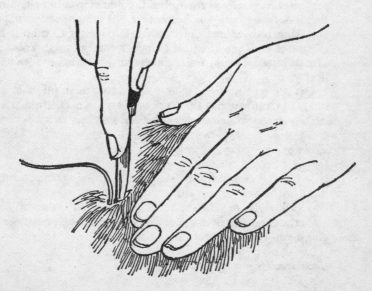

74 Fits (Convulsions)

Causes

The cause of a fit cannot be diagnosed from the type of fit or by its severity.

A fit can be the result of a variety of causes, such as epilepsy, a virus, worms, teething problems; or can be the sequel to a very high fever. With very young puppies, it can be caused by something as simple as overexcitement.

Symptoms

Fits take several forms, all of them violent and frightening.

The fit usually begins with the dog shaking its head.

This is followed by champing of the jaws, salivation, incoordination, screaming and the involuntary passage of urine and faeces.

Then the dog may fall on its side and make running movements.

The action of the jaws converts the saliva into a viscid froth, causing the dog to foam at the mouth (often terrifying those who should be helping).

Treatment (practical)

The only thing you can do for a dog which is having a fit is *prevent it from hurting itself*. And the first step is to make sure that it does not hurt *you*. Remember, the most affectionate pet is a dangerous animal during a fit. Do not try to calm it by petting or stroking. It will not do your dog any good. You will just be bitten. Do not waste time talking to the dog: it cannot hear you.

Get some blankets or pillows and throw them into a closet or small room without furniture or sharp corners. If possible, darken the room. Then move the dog into this padded area.

Technique for moving large dogs

(i)   Get behind the dog.

(ii)   Grab it firmly by the skin of the neck, just behind the head, with one hand on either side.

(iii)   Drag the dog to the room or closet put it inside and close the door. Check in ten minutes to see if the fit has passed, and if you can safely get the dog to a vet.

Technique for moving smaller, more agile dogs

(i)   Get behind the dog.

(ii)   Grab the scruff of the neck with one hand.

(iii)   With your other hand, grab both of the dog's back legs and stretch them (see illustration).

Once the animal is in a safe room, leave it alone. The fit will pass. It may take five minutes, it could take thirty minutes; but eventually the fit will pass. When it does, allow the dog to rest quietly.

Further treatment will depend upon the cause of the fit. Without medical training one can only make a guess, not a diagnosis.

The fit may have been caused by epilepsy, a virus, by worms, teething, or as the sequel to a very high fever. With very young puppies, it could have been caused by something as simple as overexcitement.

All you can do is deal with the immediate situation. Prevent the dog from hurting itself. Further treatment must be left to the vet.

---

75   Fleas

Fleas, like taxes, are a perennial problem for dog owners. Fleas not only cause your dog intense irritation and discomfort, they also carry tapeworm eggs, so get rid of them.

Your dog's fleas may bite you, but you will be glad to know that it is only in passing; dog fleas will not live on humans.

Technique for moving a small dog having a fit   **13**

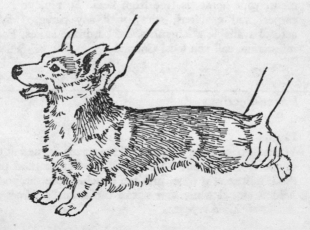

Description

1 When grooming your dog, if you notice small, reddish, flat creatures running through the hair, your dog has fleas.

2 When the hair of a dog with fleas is parted, it will look as though tiny particles of black grit have been scattered through the hairs. These are flea droppings.

Treatment

(i) Give the dog a bath with a shampoo containing selenium, such as Selsun (available at chemists) every three days for two weeks.

(ii) On the days when the dog is not being bathed, powder it thoroughly with either pyrethrum or derris powder (also available at chemists and most pet shops).

(iii) During the flea season, which varies with locale, the dog should wear a flea collar (available from pet shops). Change the collar at regular intervals of three to five weeks.

(iv) Supplement baths and powderings with patent aerosol sprays, which kill fleas on contact (available from pet shops). Dust liberal amounts of flea powder on and around the dog's sleeping area.

Treatment (*puppies*)

Puppies under eight weeks of age should not be powdered.

Simply bath them in a diluted selenium shampoo. Make sure that you wash off all the shampoo after bathing. Dry them well.

While de-fleaing the dog, be sure that the animal's environment, your home, is free from fleas. To remove fleas from carpets and cushions, spray with any patented fly-killing aerosol available at chemists and hardware stores. For heavy infestation, call you local Council.

---

76   Force-Feeding

Fluids

When force-feeding a fluid, pull the pouch formed at the side of the dog's lips out a little with your finger, and pour the fluid, a little at a time, into the pouch. Close the pouch and hold it closed while you stroke the animal's throat until it swallows. Then repeat.

Solid Food

Break the food into small pellets and feed them exactly as you would administer a tablet or pill. Hold the dog's muzzle with your left hand, thumb on one side, the rest of your fingers on the other side. With the index finger of your right hand, press down on the lower incisors (front teeth). Then place the pellet far back in the dog's mouth. Hold its mouth shut. Stroke the throat until it swallows. Then begin again.

---

77   Foreign Bodies

In the Ear
Symptoms
Excessive shaking of the head. Scratching of the ear

Treatment
Most foreign bodies in the ear can be removed by pouring a little olive oil or cooking oil into the ear, then gently massaging the ear until the object is floated out.

WARNING
Do not poke anything smaller than your left elbow into the dog's ear. If you cannot remove the object by the olive oil method, take the dog to a vet (see **Acute Otitis**).

In the Eye
The foreign body may be a grass seed, a bit of grit or a grain of sand.

If the foreign body perforates the eyeball, it will cause extreme pain. Do not attempt to remove an object that has punctured the eyeball. Get the dog to a vet at once.

Symptoms
Sudden and profuse crying, but the tears flow out of *one eye only*. There will be acute irritation of that eyeball as well.

Treatment
(i) Make a saline solution (sterile solution) by adding 1 teaspoon (5 ml) cooking salt to 1 pint (500 ml) water. Bring the water to the boil. Allow time for the water to cool.
(ii) Bathe the eye liberally with this saline solution.
To bathe the eye, use an eyedropper, or saturate a wad of cotton wool with the solution and squeeze it into the eye.

(iii) Apply a soothing ophthalmic ointment (such as Golden Eye ointment, or consult your chemist) *directly on to the eyeball*.

The technique for applying the ointment is to place the thumb and index finger of the left hand above and below the affected eye. Squeeze the ointment into the corner of the eye with your right hand. Close the eyelid with the thumb and index finger of your left hand and hold it closed for a few seconds. This will spread the ointment over the whole eyeball.

If the dog insists on scratching, even after treatment, then the foreign body may still be in the eye. Take the dog to a vet.

One of the most common causes of foreign objects in the eye is the result of dogs hanging their heads out of car windows. Exposure of the eyes to high winds can be injurious, so roll up the window when you take your dog for a car ride.

In the Foot
Foreign bodies in the foot pads are usually pieces of glass that cut the pad and work their way into the paw, or pieces of grit that have found their way into existing breaks.

Symptoms
Acute lameness. Hobbling. The dog may chew at its foot.

In later stages, the affected foot will be hot and swollen and the skin of the pad will be shiny.

There may be pus coming from the hole caused by the foreign object.

Treatment
You will need an assistant to hold the dog while you operate.
(i) Get the dog into a good light.
(ii) Sterilize a needle by boiling it for twenty minutes and then carefully probe the hole until the foreign object is visible.
(iii) With the aid of tweezers, remove it.
(iv) Dress the wound.
(v) Use the same technique you would use for removing a splinter from your own foot.
(vi) If probing with the needle does not remove the foreign body, then prepare a kaolin *poultice* and apply it to the affected pad for two days. This should draw out the object or at least make it easier for you to remove it with your needle and tweezers.

Kaolin poultice

Kaolin may be purchased at the chemist's. Prepare the *poultice* by heating the kaolin clay and pouring it on to a wad of cotton wool. Do not apply it if it is too hot. Judge this by applying it to the back of your own hand. It should be very hot but not so hot that it burns you. Then bandage it on to the foot for three to four hours, and repeat. Use plenty of elasto-plast when bandaging to prevent the dog from chewing it off. But if the animal still insists on chewing at it, use an Elizabethan Collar. See **Elizabethan Collar.**

78 Fractures

A fracture is the medical term used to describe a broken bone.

Simple fracture

If only bone is broken and there is no communicating wound between the fracture and the skin, it is called a *simple fracture*.

Compound fracture

If the skin over the fracture site is broken, thus making it possible for germs to enter from the external wound, it is called a *compound fracture*.

Complicated fracture

This type of fracture may be either simple or compound, but there is also injury to some internal organ, blood-vessel, nerve or joint.

An originally simple fracture can be turned into a compound or complicated fracture by allowing the injured animal com-plete freedom of movement or by carelessness or ignorance on the part of the owner.

When rendering first aid for fractures, there are two main objectives:

1 Guard against further injury.
2 Reduce the pain the dog is suffering.

General treatment

(i) Injured dogs must be approached and handled with great caution. An animal in pain is dangerous to you and to itself. See **Restraint.**

(ii) If a fracture is suspected, handle the limb or broken bone as little as possible.

(iii)   Make the dog as comfortable and as warm as possible. Administer aspirin to control the pain. Give 300 mg for small dogs, and up to 1500 mg for large dogs. Administer once only. See **Tablets and Pills: Techniques of Administration.**

(iv)   Basic first aid is aimed at providing a support for the fractured bone. To accomplish this a splint is applied to the fractured bone, at the point of the fracture. The splint is, in effect, a vice, between which the broken bones are held in place until professional help is obtained. (To make a splint, see below).

(v)   Do not attempt to reduce fractures and reset broken bones in the correct position. This will cause extreme pain and should be done only under anaesthetic.

(vi)   Seek professional assistance as soon as possible. Splints applied by dog owners must be considered as temporary measures and to be attempted only when a vet is not available.

Causes

Most fractures are caused by accidents, but occasionally they occur spontaneously when a bone is undergoing pathological change, such as calcium deficiency or bone cancer.

Symptoms

The fractures most commonly seen in dogs are fractures involving the legs.

1   Acute and profound lameness of the affected leg.
2   Considerable pain.
3   Possibly swelling at the site of the fracture.
4   Possibly shortening of the fractured limb.
5   When the dog is lifted off the ground, the affected limb very often will swing freely but abnormally.

As a general rule, some or all of these symptoms will be seen in a dog with a leg fracture.

Fractures of the bones of the foot

A fractured foot will be very swollen, very sore, and will have a number of cuts on it. Obviously, the dog will have to be seen by a vet. If one is not immediately available, then treat by bandaging. See **Bandaging**. Get professional help at the first opportunity.

Fractures of the jaws

Fractures of the jaws are frequently seen in dogs hit by cars or which have fallen from a considerable height. When a dog falls from a height, the front legs sometimes give way and the chin hits the ground, causing a fracture of the lower jaw.

If the dog falls from an even greater height, a fracture of the upper jaw, which appears as a split in the roof of the mouth, may be seen.

Symptoms
1 If the lower jaw has been fractured, it usually hangs slightly open. This is accompanied by profuse salivation, dribbling and drooling.
2 Closer examination will reveal a pronounced split in the middle of the front teeth, or a split in the roof of the mouth.

Treatment
If the jaw is hanging open, tie a light dressing under the chin to support it and around the back of the head (tie the dressing off behind the ears) to give support to the jaw. Then get the injured dog to a vet.

Fractures of the limbs (lower)
These are among the most common fractures seen. The dog will be unable to put the injured foot on the ground, and as it hobbles along, the leg will swing freely. If professional help is not available within twenty-four hours, fractures of the lower leg should be supported by a simple splint.

Fractures of the limbs (upper)
These are extremely difficult to splint and should be left alone until professional help is available.

To make a splint
Tie a tape muzzle around the dog's mouth. Lay the dog on its side, injured leg uppermost. Then place the injured leg on a thin piece of wood, or corrugated cardboard, and tape the leg to the wood with strips of elastoplast.

This splint is intended to simply correct excessive movement and not as a permanent repair, or as a replacement of a vet's services.

Fractures of the pelvis
A dog with a fractured pelvis will be unable to support any weight on either of its hind legs.

However, since a dog with both hind legs fractured or with a spinal fracture will also be unable to stand, the definite diagnosis of a fractured pelvis can only be made by means of an X-ray.

Treatment
A fracture of the pelvis does not require splinting.

Keep the dog in a confined space until a vet has been consulted.

Fractures of the skull
Seen after road accidents, falls, blows. They may cause incoordination, unconsciousness or nosebleeds.

If a fracture of the skull is suspected, (only from an X-ray can a definite diagnosis be made) *do not bandage the skull*; it may be a depressed fracture and bandaging would only make it worse.

If there is bleeding, use simple first aid to stop it. Be very gentle, especially in the area of the skull.

Give no drugs or fluids until a vet is seen.

---

79 Frostbite

In this condition, destruction of the tissues is caused by exposure to severe cold.

The parts of the body most often frostbitten are the nose, toes, tip of the ears and top of the tail.

Symptoms
In mild cases, the frostbitten skin becomes cold and white. There is a loss of hair around the affected parts.

In more severe cases, the loss of hair is followed by redness and localized pain.

In even more serious cases, the area remains sore, sensitive to the touch, swells, then shrivels. Finally, the skin around the affected area sloughs away, leaving an open, weeping surface.

Treatment
In mild cases, increase the circulation of blood to the frostbitten area by rubbing the area briskly with your hand.

Then apply camphorated oil or oil of wintergreen.

If the dog is very uncomfortable, administer an analgesic such as aspirin (300 mg for small dogs, and up to 1500 mg for large dogs), once only in a twenty-four hour period. See **Tablets and Pills: Techniques of Administration.**

In the most extreme cases, amputation may be necessary (see **Gangrene**).

---

80 Gangrene

The term is applied to either:
1 A specific localized condition.
2 A portion of the body in which the tissues are dead because the blood supply to that portion has been restricted.

Infection symptoms
When gangrene is due to an infection, it usually follows bite wounds, especially on the feet. These wounds become infected. If the infection is left untreated, it may become gangrenous. A bite around the area of the wrist can become infected and the lack of blood causes gangrene of the toes.

The infection develops fairly rapidly and the infected area becomes swollen, foul-smelling, and gives off a bubbly discharge.

Treatment
Professional. Get the dog to a vet.

Blood restriction symptoms
Gangrene caused by restriction of the blood supply to a part of the body is seen when bandages are applied too tightly or when a tourniquet is left on too long. It also occurs (far too frequently) when children put elastic bands around the dog's neck, paws or scrotum.

Treatment
(i) Remove the source of constriction.
(ii) Clean the area with hydrogen peroxide, Savlon or just soap and water and apply warm compresses to encourage the blood to circulate again.
(iii) Get professional help.

---

81 Gastroenteritis

Gastroenteritis is a general term for an infection of the stomach and intestines which is characterized by vomiting and diarrhoea.

Symptoms (Fever Stage)
The dog loses its appetite, mopes about, and shows no enthusiasm.

The animal may also run a high fever and may show signs of abdominal pain. Dogs with abdominal pain often lie with their rear legs up and their front legs extended. Also, they tend to seek out cold places, like cement floors, to lie on and they show signs of restlessness.

A dog with a *high fever* will have dull eyes, a worn expression, a dry hot nose, a dry coat. Quite simply, the dog looks ill.

Symptoms (Vomiting Stage)
The next stage is characterized by continual vomiting. Initially, the vomit is white and frothy, then it becomes yellow. In advanced stages, it may become bloodstained. During this vomiting stage, the dog will be very thirsty. It will drink and then vomit, setting up a drink-vomit cycle.

Symptoms (Diarrhoea Stage)
Once the vomiting stage has been established, diarrhoea usually begins. About twenty-four hours later, the diarrhoea becomes blood-stained.

Treatment
Withhold food and water for up to twenty-four hours, until you have had professional advice.

---

82   Gingivitis

Gingivitis is an infection of the gums which appears at the margin of tooth and gum. It is often seen in association with *tartar*.

Symptoms
1   The classic symptom of this infection is a red line along the gum, above the tooth or teeth.
2   Halitosis.

Treatment
Since gingivitis is often caused by general infections of the mouth and throat as well as by more specific infections, the exact cause of the condition must be identified and eliminated.

The gingivitis itself is easily treated by applying a solution made from hydrogen peroxide, 20 vol (obtainable from chemists). Use 1 part hydrogen peroxide to 3 parts water.

Swab the gums with this solution every three hours. If the condition has not cleared up after three days of treatment, professional help should be sought.

---

83   Glucose

This is a type of sugar, which provides quick energy, to be given when the dog is weak and apathetic. Simply sprinkle the powder on the food or put it into the water.

Substitute
If a glucose powder is not available, a substitute mixture can be made by adding 2 tablespoons of sugar to 1 pint (500 ml) water and stirring until the sugar has dissolved.

---

84   Grass Seeds

In the summer and early autumn, the drying seeds of barley grasses can cause a good deal of pain by penetrating between the dog's toes, down its ears, in its eyes or up its nose. If left untreated, the seeds, which are barbed like fish-hooks, will migrate inwards, eventually producing discharging wounds.

Ears
Symptoms
A grass seed down the ear will cause very painful symptoms. The dog will rub its face on the ground, paw at its ears and walk with its head on one side as though attempting to dislodge something.

Treatment
Pour warm olive oil or cooking oil into the ear and massage the ear gently to float the seed out.

Eyes
Symptoms
Profuse crying from *one eye only*. Extreme irritation of the eye. It will become very red and obviously painful.

Treatment

If the seed has not penetrated the eyeball, wash it out of the eye with a saline solution. (See **Saline Solution**). If the seed has penetrated the eyeball, *do not attempt to remove it*; get the dog to a vet.

Nose

Symptoms

A grass seed up the nose will cause severe bouts of sneezing.

Treatment

Get a good light and shine it up the dog's nose. If the seed is visible, it may be removed with tweezers. If you do use tweezers, be very careful not to injure the delicate nasal lining. If your dog is difficult to control, you will need an assistant to hold the animal (see **Restraint**). And if the dog is very difficult, do not attempt to put anything up its nose. Leave that to the vet.

Between the Toes

Symptoms

A grass seed lodged between the toes produces pustules which may cause the dog to limp. If left untreated, the seed will work its way into the foot and produce breaks in the skin which may be confused with those of interdigital cysts.

Treatment

If you can see the seed, use a pair of tweezers to pull it out.

---

85   Grooming

Most dogs groom themselves, but the wise dog owner does not leave the job entirely to the animal. The act of grooming not only helps the dog keep clean, but it establishes a physical rapport between dog and owner. This rapport will stand the owner in good stead on those occasions when it is necessary to handle the dog in order to administer first aid.

Healthy dogs will do their best to keep their coats clean, but even the most zealous dog is unable to keep up with the city's accumulation of grime. It is well to remember that our dogs live in a world 6 in (15 cm) to 3 ft (1 m) in height, about level with car exhaust pipes.

City dogs should be bathed once a month. Small dogs can

be put in a tub; larger dogs, with an aversion to baths, should be washed with a hose. If it is a large dog living in a small flat, where hosing is not practical, then the tub will have to be used. In this case, an assistant will be very helpful. Also, be prepared to get wet. Even though many dogs, like young children, dislike baths, they can be bathed against their wishes. Be determined, be firm; know what you are going to do and get on with it.

WARNING
If the dog's grooming is neglected, and its coat is allowed to become filthy and matted, the dog will develop a predisposition to skin diseases.

Grooming and sick animals
(i) The importance of grooming as a factor in nursing, contributing to the dog's well-being, cannot be overemphasized. Sick dogs may neglect their grooming. Sick dogs have an excuse; their owners do not.
(ii) Apart from the coat, keep the eyes, nose, ears and around the mouth clean by wiping regularly with a little diluted Cetavlon on cotton wool. Use 1 teaspoon (5 ml) Cetavlon to 10 teaspoons (50 ml) water.
(iii) A dog with diarrhoea will develop a sore anus. Treat this soreness by applying an antiseptic cream, eg zinc and castor-oil cream, or cold cream.
If it is not desirable to bath a dog in water, there are several 'dry bath' preparations available. These are in the form of powder which is dusted into the dog's coat and then brushed out. Unfortunately, dry shampoos, while convenient, simply do not do an adequate job. While dry shampoos are better than nothing, they are not nearly so effective as wet shampoos.

All dogs should be brushed daily. Long-haired dogs should also be combed, and any knots of tangled hair that do not comb out should be cut out with scissors.

Long-haired breeds which are not brushed regularly may develop hair balls in their stomach, from the accumulation of loose hair they swallow while grooming themselves (see **Hair Balls**).

86   Haemorrhage from the Ear

Often seen after fights or road accidents. Bleeding may be

coming from the ear flap or from inside the ear.

Treatment
Whether the bleeding originates from the ear flap or from the ear itself, the treatment is the same:
(i)   Pack the ear canal with cotton wool (not too much, just enough to fill the ear without overpacking).
(ii)   Bandage the ear (see **Bandaging the Ears**). The bandage may be left on for three to four days.

WARNING
If left untreated, bleeding from the ear may develop into a middle ear infection.

87   Haemorrhage from the Vagina

While some slight bleeding from the vagina is normal during heat periods, heavy bleeding requires immediate professional assistance.

Treatment
(i)   See **Shock**; also **Abortion.**
(ii)   Keep the bitch warm and quiet until professional help is available.

88   Hair Balls

Cause
Hair balls usually occur in long-haired dogs which are not being adequately groomed.

When the dog licks itself, it swallows those loose hairs which have not been brushed and combed out of its coat.

In most instances, these hairs are vomited up; but if this does not happen, then the hair accumulates in the dog's stomach.

Symptoms
1   Soon after eating, the dog vomits.
2   Straining to pass a motion.
3   Constipation.

Treatment
In most instances, the dog will eventually pass the hair ball. In acute cases, where there is continual vomiting after eating, administer 2 tablespoons (50 ml) liquid paraffin.

Prevention
The best method of prevention is the most obvious one. Brush and comb your pet regularly (see **Grooming**).

89   Hair Loss (Moulting)

A certain degree of moulting is natural, occurring twice a year, during the spring and autumn. If the dog loses large amounts of hair at other times, check first to make sure that the animal is being properly and regularly groomed. If regular grooming has been carried out, then this loss of hair must be considered abnormal.

Causes
Moulting may be due to thyroid deficiency; chronic nephritis; malnutrition; hormone deficiency; fatty acid deficiency.

General treatment
(i)   Bath and groom the dog. Use a selenium-based shampoo, eg Selsun.
(ii)   Add corn oil to the moulting dog's diet. 1 teaspoon (5 ml) a week for a small dog, up to 5 tablespoons (125 ml) a week for a large dog, should improve the condition.

90   Heat Periods (Oestrus Cycle)

'Heat' or 'season' is the term used to describe the time when the female dog will mate. It is during this period that pregnancy may occur.

A bitch's first season usually occurs when she is between six and nine months old. Bitches are capable of conceiving throughout their lives. They are never too old to have a litter. Bitches come into heat twice a year. This regular cyclic progression is interrupted only by pregnancy.

Each heat lasts approximately eighteen days and may be divided into two stages.

First stage of heat

1   During the first stage the bitch's vulva swells noticeably and the owner will observe a blood-tinged discharge.
2   The bitch becomes attractive to and attracts the attention of dogs, but during this first stage she will not be interested in mating.
3   Her appetite and drinking habits may become capricious. This first stage lasts about nine days after the signs of heat first appear. Then the second stage occurs.

Second stage of heat

1   During this stage the bitch is capable of conceiving.
2   The discharge from the vulva is straw-coloured and free from blood.
3   She will readily accept any dog.
4   She develops wanderlust and, if allowed, will stray from home in the company of male followers.

---

91   Heat Stroke

Cause

Prolonged exposure to a source of heat, or overcrowding. The classic cases of heat stroke are seen when dogs are left in cars on hot days or packed into travelling cages that are too small.

Breeds with heavy coats are particularly susceptible to heat stroke. And, of course, the condition is aggravated by lack of water.

Symptoms

Panting, dullness, stumbling, sweating through the foot pads.

In the later stages the dog runs a very high temperature, up to 110°F (43°C), falls into a coma and finally dies.

Treatment

(i)   Give the dog water *immediately*.
(ii)   Cool the dog by hosing and sponging with cold water and by applying ice packs all over the body, with special attention to the head and chest.
(iii)   Further administration of glucose and water. Mix 4 tablespoons glucose with 1 pint (500 ml) water. Give 4 oz (100 ml) of the solution for small dogs, and up to 1 pint (500 ml) for large dogs.

Hernia

A hernia is the protrusion of internal tissues through a natural opening, such as the navel or the inguinal canal in the groin, which would normally close in the course of growth. There are four types of hernia: inguinal, scrotal, traumatic and umbilical. However, the traumatic hernia is not a true hernia.

Inguinal Hernia
A swelling in the groin which continues to grow. Most bitches have tiny inguinal hernias.

Treatment
Surgical.

Scrotal Hernia
A swelling of the scrotum.

Symptoms
This swelling is particularly noticeable after the dog has eaten a heavy meal. There may be discomfort and in severe cases acute pain and possible strangulation of the bowel.

Treatment
The only remedy for this form is surgical.

EMERGENCY
If the pain is obviously acute, professional assistance must be sought without delay. The danger comes from possible strangulation of the bowel, and this constitutes an emergency.

Traumatic Hernia
This occurs after accidents and requires immediate professional treatment. In fact, it is not a true hernia, but a rupture. See **Injuries to the Abdomen with Intestinal Protrusion**.

Umbilical Hernia
Seen fairly frequently in puppies.

Symptoms
There is a small protrusion of intestinal fat visible at the navel.

Treatment
This form of hernia is not often serious, providing the bit of

fat protruding is pliable and small, $\frac{1}{4}$ in ($\frac{1}{2}$ cm) or less. The puppy grows, but the protrusion remains small. So leave it alone.

If the protruding portion is larger than that, the pup should be taken to a vet for minor surgery.

---

93   Hiccups

Causes
Puppies which bolt their food often get hiccups.

They also get hiccups if their stomachs are empty.

Occasionally the adult dog will also develop hiccups.

Treatment for adult dogs
The condition is not serious and usually disappears of its own accord. However, if the hiccups do persist for more than half an hour, administer 1 tablespoon (25 ml) milk of magnesia.

Puppies
There is no need to worry about hiccups in puppies. If the hiccups appear to be causing the pup distress, put a little olive oil on your finger and gently rub the pup's abdomen to induce burping.

---

94   Humans Bitten by Dogs

Treatment
(i)   Wash the bite with soap and cooled boiled water.

(ii)   Rinse the soap off.

(iii)   Cover the bite with a clean bandage.

(iv)   Visit your doctor, or the casualty department of the local hospital. Remember, all animal bites are contaminated and, if it is a deep bite, an anti-tetanus injection should be given.

---

95   Hysteria

Certain individual dogs and certain breeds seem to be hysteria-prone.

Description
Hysteria usually begins with a long bout of barking. The dog

behaves as though it were terrified, and runs about yelping wildly and bouncing off walls and furniture. As with fits, there may be involuntary passage of urine and faeces. The hysterical dog will not respond to commands. It will try to evade capture and it will bite, if it can. Handle it carefully (see **Restraint**).

Treatment
Treat a hysterical dog as you would treat a dog having a fit or convulsion. Get it into a quiet, darkened empty room or closet where it cannot hurt itself.

The line between hysteria and a fit is very thin and a hysterical dog, if not promptly attended to, may very well drift over that line and into a full-fledged fit.

---

96   Inability to give Milk (Agalactia)

Agalactia is the inability of an animal to give milk.

Causes
The cause can be hereditary; it can be the result of a hormonal imbalance; or the sequel to an infection or breast cancer. Agalactia often occurs with bitches giving birth to their first litters.

Symptoms
The behaviour of the puppies is your best indication of agalactia. If they are not getting their milk, they will scream and whine with hunger and will be restless and fretful, just as a human baby would be. The mother, however, will appear quite normal.

Treatment
(i)   Apply warm compresses to the mother's mammary glands for ten minutes at a time, four or five times a day.
(ii)   Gentle massage of the mammary glands with olive oil may stimulate and restore their function.
(iii)   Hormone therapy with pituitary hormones. This treatment, which requires the services of a vet, may induce milk production within twenty-four hours.
(iv)   These treatments, of course, apply only to the mother. Meanwhile, while waiting for the production of milk, the new-born puppies must be fed every two hours (see **Orphan Puppies**).

97   Inflammation of the Tongue (Glossitis)

Causes

Numerous. Most of them serious. The inflammation could be the result of chronic interstitial nephritis, corrosive poisons, fish-hooks or other trauma.

Symptoms

Severe dribbling, accompanied by loss of appetite and halitosis.

Open the dog's mouth and look for a raw, red, sore circular patch or patches. These are ulcers on the tongue.

In later stages there is a foul, brownish drainage from the corner of the mouth which drips down the chest and paws. Look for drainage stains on your dog's chest and paws.

Treatment

(i)   The dog's mouth must be kept as clean as possible by washing it with a solution of dilute hydrogen peroxide or very dilute Savlon.

(ii)   The solution is made by mixing 1 teaspoon (5 ml) Savlon per 1 pint (500 ml) water, or 1 teaspoon (5 ml) of 20 vol hydrogen peroxide (available at any chemist's) to 3 teaspoons (15 ml) water. This solution should be administered every two hours. If there is no improvement after twenty-four hours, contact a vet.

98   Injections

While it is not usual for dog owners to administer injections, there are occasional situations such as diabetes or certain long courses of antibiotic treatment when knowledge of the technique can be very useful.

The subcutaneous injection is an injection under the skin, as opposed to the intravenous injection which is directly into a vein. The subcutaneous injection is relatively simple to administer and completely painless.

When administering an injection, act with confidence and self-assurance. If you are hesitant and unsure of yourself, the dog will sense it and the process will be that much more difficult.

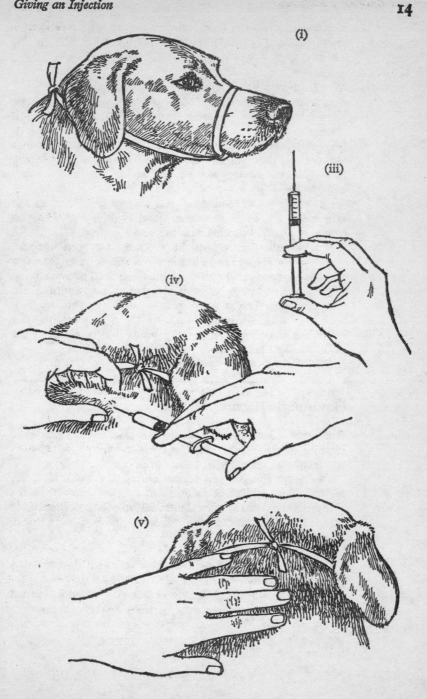

(i)

(iii)

(iv)

(v)

Technique

(i) If there is someone available, ask him to hold your dog for you. If there is a possibility that the dog might bite, tape its muzzle.

(ii) Saturate a pad of cotton wool with alcohol and swab the skin around the scruff of the neck, where the injection will be administered. Do not make a great show of this, or you will alarm the dog. A quick rub with the cotton wool is sufficient.

(iii) After filling the syringe, hold it point uppermost and slowly press the plunger until all the air is out of the syringe.

(iv) Hold the syringe at the base, between your index finger and thumb. With your other hand, lift a fold of skin at the scruff of the neck into a cone, and slip the needle under the skin below the cone. Press the plunger. Keep the needle as nearly as possible parallel with the skin's surface.

(v) When the contents of the syringe have been injected, withdraw the syringe and rub the site of the injection for a few seconds to make certain that the fluid has been dispersed.

(vi) If an assistant is not available, there is no great problem. You can easily hold most animals by the scruff of the neck with one hand, while administering the injection with your other hand. And, by holding the animal by the scruff of the neck, you also minimize the danger of being bitten.

---

99 Injuries to the Abdomen with Intestinal Protrusion (Traumatic Hernia)

Dogs involved in fights or a variety of accidents (road accidents, jumping on fences, etc) may tear their abdominal wall to such an extent that the internal organs protrude.

Obviously, this is a very serious emergency, but it need not be fatal. The real danger comes from the possibility of haemorrhage, shock, or from accidental self-mutilation. Immediate first aid can prevent this.

Treatment

(i) Assess the damage. If there is no vet available, then be prepared to do more than just bandage the wound.

(ii) Calm the animal. Try not to touch the wound more than you have to. If the protruding portions of the intestines are dirty, they should be washed gently in boiled water, which has been cooled. To wash, simply pour the water over the protruding part of the intestines.

(iii)   If just a small portion of the intestines protrudes, *gently* try to push it back into the dog's abdomen through the wound.
(iv)   Place a pad over the wound and then bandage the pad around the dog's body.
(v)   Treat for shock if necessary.
(vi)   Seek professional help immediately.

100   Interdigital Cyst

A distressing condition often seen in Alsatians, boxers, Labradors and terriers, the cause of which is unknown.

Symptoms
A shiny red swelling between the toes. This swelling is sore and painful and it continues to swell until it bursts, liberating a clear reddish fluid.

Treatment
(i)   Soften the affected part by bathing it four times a day in a warm saline solution until the swelling bursts. Continue bathing until the wound heals. This usually takes about a week.
(ii)   Then paint the area with a solution of 2 per cent phenol, using an eyedropper or paintbrush. Be careful not to use too much phenol; it is caustic and can be painful. (Phenol is available from chemists).
(iii)   In very serious cases, surgical treatment and a course of antibiotics may be necessary.

101   Internal Bleeding (Internal Haemorrhage)

Causes
Road accidents, falls and eating coagulant poisons (Warfarin, mouse and rat poison) can produce internal bleeding.

Symptoms
The overall symptoms are the same as those in cases of severe shock.
1   The animal exhibits pronounced weakness and heavy panting.
2   The pulse rate is very fast but weak.
3   The mucous membranes around the lips and nose are pale.

4   The dog's paws will be cold.

Treatment
There is no first aid treatment for this condition. The only certain way of controlling the bleeding is surgical.

EMERGENCY
If these symptoms are observed, *do not waste time*. Wrap the dog in a blanket and get it to a vet.
Have someone telephone the vet first, if possible, so that he can have the necessary preparations ready for you.

---

102   Irretractable Penis (Paraphimosis)

In this condition the penis protrudes from the sheath instead of sliding back into place.

Causes
1   The sheath opening is too small.
2   Hypersexuality.

Treatment
(i)   Apply warm olive oil to the shaft of the penis. Then, gently manipulate it back into the sheath.
(ii)   With smaller dogs, simply plunge them into a cold bath. The penis should retract automatically.

---

103   Jelly-Fish Stings

Symptoms
These vary according to the species of jelly-fish and the site of the sting. Generally speaking, if the dog, after swimming in the sea, exhibits extreme and obvious pain, treat for jelly-fish sting.

Treatment
(i)   Relieve the pain. Begin by making certain that there are no tentacles of the jelly-fish still clinging to the dog's skin. (Be careful when removing tentacles; they can still sting!)
(ii)   If the dog is suffering more than mild discomfort, administer half a tablet to two tablets of aspirin, depending upon *body weight*.

(iii) Local applications of soothing solutions such as olive oil, sodium bicarbonate, are helpful.

(iv) If available, a solution of dilute ammonia (1 part ammonia to 10 parts water) applied at once will prevent most of the painful results of the sting.

Severe cases

In severe cases, naturally the symptoms will be much more dramatic and much more serious. The dog owner will not have the necessary medicines for alleviating the toxic effects of the sting. So, in these extreme cases, he had better concern himself with any symptoms of shock that may appear. See **Shock.**

Keep the dog warm. Give it a solution of 4 tablespoons glucose to 1 pint (500 ml) water. Give 4 oz (100 ml) of this solution for small dogs, and up to 1 pint (500 ml) for large dogs. See **Force-Feeding.**

If the dog stops breathing, artificial respiration should be administered. See **Artificial Respiration.**

In these extreme cases, every effort should be made to get the dog to a vet.

---

104 Kidney Failure, Renal Failure (Chronic Interstitial Nephritis)

This condition is frequently seen in elderly dogs (seven years or older), following an infection of *leptospira canicola* (leptospirosis) in particular.

Symptoms

1 The dog is constantly thirsty. Its physical condition deteriorates. The coat is dull and there are skin eruptions.
2 As the condition progresses, the dog vomits frequently and suffers from diarrhoea and excessive urination and thirst.
3 The dog's breath is bad.
4 The urine is pale and watery.

The disease occurs in two forms:

In the first form, called the 'compensated' form, the dog drinks excessively and is able to flush the poison through its kidneys.

In the second form, called the 'decompensated' form, the dog is unable to flush the poisons out of its body and may die of accumulated poisons (toxaemia and uraemia).

Treatment
(i) The dog must be given as much clean water as it can drink. Make sure that its water bowl is always full.
(ii) Put your dog on a low protein diet of the white meat from boned chicken and fish, or on the proprietary nephritis diet available from the vet.
(iii) Antibiotic treatment may be helpful, but this must be left to the discretion of the vet.

105 Lameness

Also see **Limping**. In cases of severe lameness, the dog owner should not rely upon his own diagnosis if professional help is available. Improperly diagnosed fractures and dislocations can lead to severe complications.

As a general rule, in diagnosing causes of sudden lameness:
1 If the dog is severely lame and the limb is free-swinging, then the leg is probably fractured.
2 If there is displacement, that is if the leg is not in its normal position, the leg may be dislocated.
3 If the affected limb is neither free-swinging nor displaced, a strain or sprain may be suspected.
4 A cut or foreign body (piece of glass, splinter, etc) will also cause lameness.
More gradual and more permanent forms of lameness may be encountered with the elderly dog, caused by arthritis or neoplasms (cancerous growths). In such cases, simple analgesics may help.

106 Lead Clips Caught in the Flesh

Occasionally, when a lead clip is being attached to a dog's collar, the clip ends up attached to the loose folds of the dog's neck. It may also become attached to the web between the toes. If the clip is deeply imbedded in the skin, do not try to take it off the way you got it on. First apply a tape muzzle (see **Restraint**). Then cut off the back of the clip with a hacksaw or wire-clippers. If you do not have the tools, try the nearest garage. They will have wire-cutters.

Prevention

Do not use lead clips which are shaped like a question mark. Use the types with jointed action.

---

107 Leptospirosis

WARNING
This disease is highly contagious and can be transmitted from dogs to people.

Description
This is a bacterial disease and not due to a virus. It may respond to specific antibiotic therapy once the disease has been identified. The incubation period is from five to fifteen days.

Cause
Basically, the infection comes from contact with infected urine, which is why puppies of both sexes, and male dogs, catch leptospirosis far more often than bitches, which tend to be more discreet in their urinating habits.

Symptoms
1 The dog is dull, lethargic.
2 The animal loses its appetite, but becomes very thirsty.
3 The abdomen is sore.
4 The dog moves slowly and with evident pain.
5 The dog may show signs of jaundice. Its eyes, gums, tongue may have a yellowish caste.
6 The body temperature may rise as high as 106°F (41°C).
7 There is severe diarrhoea, some vomiting.
8 The animal's eyes are red and sore.

Treatment
(i)   Professional treatment, if at all possible. The specific drug for this condition is streptomycin, which must be given by a vet.
(ii)   The only home treatment is that of dealing with the symptoms as they arise. These symptoms include thirst, diarrhoea, vomiting (see **Excessive Drinking**).
(iii)   Hygiene is essential. Owners must not forget that they and their family can catch this disease from their dog and must act accordingly. Wash your hands after touching the dog. Keep

the dog out of the room you eat in. Sprinkle disinfectant in or around your house, wherever the dog urinates.

Prognosis
If the disease is recognized and the treatment initiated early on, there is an excellent chance of the dog's recovering.

But once jaundice has begun, the outlook is less optimistic.

---

108 Lice

Even though animal lice will not live on humans for very long, they carry disease and cause intense irritation, which may lead to complications and must not be neglected.

Description
Lice are flat little creatures, sometimes confused with fleas. But fleas can be seen running through the dog's hair, while lice will crawl slowly, or cling to the base of the hairs.

Treatment
(i)   Shampoo and bath the dog twice a week for two weeks with a shampoo containing selenium (Selsun) or with gammexane washes. Gammexane is an insecticide, available from chemists.
(ii)   In addition to the bi-weekly shampoo, apply a solution of Benzyl benzoate lotion with 1 per cent Tetmosol (solution available at chemists) over the whole dog once a month.

WARNING
When treating puppies (under six months) do not use the Benzyl benzoate solution. Just use the shampoo once a week.

---

109 Lightning Strike

Dogs, when sheltering under trees or in close contact with metallic objects, are occasionally struck by lightning.

Symptoms
1   The dog may be burned.
2   The dog may also show signs of shock, such as incoordination or even paralysis.

Treatment
(i)   Treat for shock. See **Shock.**
(ii) Treat the burns.
(iii) Administer a simple stimulant, such as caffeine (caffeine tablets are available from most chemists), strong tea or coffee. Also administer glucose and water. See **Force-Feeding.**

---

110   Limping

Causes
There are several possible causes for dogs limping. If the cause is in the foot, the dog may lick the offending paw.

Examine the paw
The first thing to do is to get the dog into a good light and then carefully examine the paw for thorns, tacks, or small cuts. You will find that it is easier to do this when the paw is wet; then the hair lies flat and the thorn or cut is more readily seen.

If it is not a thorn or a cut that is causing the limp, look for a cracked pad. You may not be able to see the cracks, so gently palpate the pad with your thumb. A cracked pad is very sensitive and pressure is painful.

Next, check for a broken claw nail. If that is what is making the dog limp, a bit of elastoplast around the broken nail will help until the nail grows back.

If none of these causes is evident, the limp may be the result of a sprain. If it is a sprain, there will be swelling, pain and localized heat.

In an elderly dog, if there is no evidence of a sprain or injury to the paw, then there is the possibility that the limp is caused by arthritis.

To decide whether or not it is arthritis, observe the dog for a few days, noting:
1   Does the dog have difficulty in rising in the morning? Does it move more easily later in the day?
2   Does a change in the weather bring a variation in the lameness?
3   Is the dog unable to jump up, manage stairs?
4   Is it lame at a walk? At a gallop?
5   Is the lameness worse with exercise?
6   Is the lameness intermittent?
If you cannot cure the lameness yourself, and you have to bring the dog to a vet, these are the questions he will ask you. You should be able to answer them.

111   Longevity

Perhaps the saddest thing about owning and loving a dog is the brevity of a dog's life span compared to our own.

Large breeds
The larger breeds have the shortest life span. Seven or eight years is a ripe old age for a Great Dane.

Small breeds
Smaller dogs are often fit at the age of thirteen or fourteen years.

112   Mange

Mange is a fairly common skin disease. It is caused by miniscule spider-like creatures, too small to be seen without a microscope.

General symptoms
1   You will observe your dog's discomfort. You will notice it biting and scratching at the infected areas.
2   Loss of hair, reddening of the skin and, occasionally, thickening or coarsening of the skin.

There are three types of mange which affect dogs
(1) demodectic mange (sometimes called 'follicular' or 'red' mange).
(2) sarcoptic mange, which is contagious to people. Demodectic and sarcoptic mange do have some general symptoms in common, but only a microscopic examination of the skin scrapings can produce a definite diagnosis.
(3) otodectic mange. See below for specific symptoms and treatment for this ear-mite infection.

Treatment (General Precautions)
(i)   Dispose of the dog's bedding.
(ii)   Use Tetmosol soap and wash the dog's collar or harness, twice a week for as long as the condition persists.
(ii)   Soap and rinse the dog's collar or harness, twice a week for as long as the condition persists.
(iii) Do not allow your dog to come into contact with other animals. When you walk the dog, keep it on the lead.

(iv)   After every treatment, use liberal amounts of soap, water and Cetavlon to thoroughly clean and disinfect the area where you have been treating the dog. Dispose of the cotton wool where no one will handle it.

(v)   Then wash your own hands.

Treatment (Specific)

(i)   Bathe the entire animal in warm water with gammexane powder (gamma benzene hexachloride) added. (The powder is available at chemists.) Use 8 oz (226 g) powder to 1 gallon (4·5 l) water. Or, use a selenium-based shampoo such as Selsun.

(ii)   Repeat this bath every five days. If there is no improvement in ten days, contact your vet.

WARNING

Never use carbolic soap or lysol to wash your dog. Dogs absorb the carbolic and lysol through their skin and though these preparations will kill the dog's mange, they may also kill the dog.

(iii)   Give relief from excessive biting and scratching, as this can cause secondary infections and other unpleasant complications. So, if the animal simply will not stop biting itself, fit it with an Elizabethan collar.

(iv)   You may also provide temporary relief by applying a soothing, cooling lotion such as calamine lotion to the irritated areas.

Otodectic Mange (Ear Mites)

Symptoms

1   Brown waxy discharge, containing crusts, can be seen in the ears.

2   There is acute irritation of the ears and the dog spends a good deal of time scratching its ears and shaking its head.

3   There may be a rattling noise from the ears when the dog shakes its head.

Treatment

In the early stages, clean the dog's ears with cotton wool dipped in a little, very dilute mixture of washing-up liquid (1 teaspoon (5 ml) washing-up liquid per ¼ pint (125 ml) water). This will get rid of the sticky wax.

Be careful, of course, when cleaning the ears, but you need not be afraid of touching the eardrum since it is well out of the way of the cotton wool. Do not use a cotton bud or Q-tip. This may damage the eardrum. After cleaning, swab the inside of the ears with a solution of Benzyl benzoate, containing I per cent Tetmosol, applied once a week for one month. This solution is available at any chemist's. No prescription is necessary.

More acute cases may require antibiotics and cortico-steroids to reduce the inflammation. Get professional advice.

---

113   Mating (Bitches)

Successful breeding
An owner who wishes to breed from his bitch should attempt to ensure that mating occurs as soon as possible after the bleeding stops. Successful breeding is most likely to occur ten to twelve days after the beginning of heat.

Control of heat
Very few owners would want their bitches to become pregnant with every heat. Fortunately, there are several methods available for preventing unwanted pregnancies.

Abortion (Mis-mating) Accidental mating can be aborted within thirty-six hours, with an injection of stilboestrol given by a vet. This injection may bring the animal on heat for a further twenty-one days.

Ovaro/Hysterectomy Removal of the uterus and ovaries to prevent heat. Its only drawback is that it is irreversible. However, it is infinitely preferable to an unwanted litter.

It is commonly and erroneously believed that a bitch will be healthy and happier if she has at least one litter before being spayed, or that it is 'cruel and unnatural' to interfere with an animal's sex life. We suggest that owners who sub-scribe to these folk prejudices examine their attitudes to be sure that they are not confusing their own sexuality with that of their pets.

Contraceptive tablets For the owner who does not wish to take the irreversible step of hysterectomy, but does not want litter after litter of puppies either, there are contraceptive tablets available from veterinary surgeons which suppress or postpone the heat.

However, these contraceptive tablets are not suitable for every bitch. Consult a vet for further information.

Post-coital problems

After mating, the dog and the bitch will remain 'tied' together for twenty minutes or so. Well-meaning but uninformed owners may attempt to separate them by throwing a pail of cold water over them, or by pulling them apart. This can cause an uncontrollable haemorrhage of the dog's penis, as well as inflicting appreciable damage to the vagina. When a pair of dogs are tied together after mating, leave them alone.

---

114   Milk Fever (Eclampsia)

This condition is seen in all breeds of dogs but it occurs more frequently in the smaller breeds, especially ones which have just had large litters.

Cause
Calcium deficiency.

Symptoms
1   Milk fever usually manifests itself just before the puppies are weaned, about five to six weeks after birth.
2   The bitch becomes very restless. She whimpers a great deal and lies with her legs extended, breathing rapidly.
3   She may lose her sense of coordination and when she tries to stand, falls over.
4   This stage is associated with a rise in body temperature up to 107°F (41°C).
5   There is dribbling, rigidity and convulsions.

WARNING
If she is in this state and is left untreated, the bitch will die.

Treatment
(i)   Treatment is simple, but it must be administered by a vet. It consists of intravenous calcium borogluconate.
(ii)   If convulsions have not started, owners can mix 4 oz (113 g) calcium borogluconate with 1 pint (500 ml) water, and give this solution by mouth until the symptoms stop or the vet arrives.

Prevention
During lactation give milk and bone-meal to the bitch. Your vet will advise quantities.
See also **Unconsciousness, Birth, Diet, Analgesics, Fits.**

115 Mis-mating (Mésalliance)

If a bitch mates with an undesirable dog, take her to a veterinary surgeon *within thirty-six hours*. An injection of stilboestrol will nullify the conception.

WARNING
Never attempt to force mating dogs apart. This could cause severe pain and haemorrhage in both animals. Besides, it is a wasted effort, since conception usually occurs within sixty seconds of penetration.

116 Mother Dog Eating Her Puppies

A bitch having her first litter should be carefully watched, for in certain instances she may attempt to eat her young. This is not as monstrous nor as abnormal as it sounds.

It may be the result of a natural fright response, but more often it is caused by a faulty placenta-eating instinct. In this case, the mother simply does not know where the placenta (afterbirth) ends and her new-born puppies begin.

If a bitch seems nervous or overprotective towards her newborn litter, or if she objects to strangers (or even family) handling her young, humour her. Keep the strangers and the rest of the family away from the pups. Of course, children are the main offenders and it is difficult to refuse them the delights of handling new-born puppies, but if the puppies' mother shows any resentment, this must be done. After all, they are *her* puppies.

117 Motion Sickness

This condition is common in dogs, especially those unaccustomed to travelling.

Symptoms
Restlessness, excessive salivation and persistent vomiting.

Treatment
(i) Before the trip, administer an animal tranquillizer such as acetyl promazine, or any of the phenothiazine derivatives. (These can be obtained from a vet.)

(ii) If animal tranquillizers are not available, preparations for human travel sickness, available from chemists, may be administered instead. Kwells, or Marzine, are both recommended. The dosage will vary with the size of the dog. But a fair estimate is one-quarter of the adult human dosage per 20 lb (9·10 kg) animal *body weight*.

Prevention
(i) Before long journeys, withhold all food for twenty-four hours, but give your dog plenty of water.
(ii) Get your dog accustomed to car travel by taking it on short car trips when possible. Also, allow the dog to spend time in the car when it is at home, stationary.

---

118 Nasal Discharge

A thick, yellowy mucus suggests distemper or one of the other canine virus diseases (see also **Sinusitis**). Obviously a vet should be consulted.
Normally, a healthy dog's nose is cold and wet. A hot, dry nose suggests fever and warrants further examination.

---

119 Neuralgia

Symptoms
1 Sudden and obvious pain.
2 The muscles of the dog's neck, back or legs, depending upon where the neuralgia is being experienced, grow very tense.
3 These attacks of neuralgia are intermittent and may last for several hours.

Treatment
(i) Keep the dog warm and allow it to rest.
(ii) An infra-red ray lamp is a great comfort to a dog suffering from neuralgia. Mount the lamp about 3 ft (1 m) over the dog's bed and leave it on all night. In the absence of an infra-red ray lamp, an electric blanket or hot water bottle is also helpful.
(iii) Administer up to two 300 mg aspirin tablets, depending upon body weight, to ease the pain.

120 Nipple Soreness

Cause
This condition is seen fairly often while the female is nursing her litter.

It is caused by the nails of the puppies pricking the soft flesh of the mother's teats.

Symptoms
1 The babies will be screaming for food.
2 The bitch's nipples will be red and cracked.

Treatment
(i) If the mother's nipples are simply sore and red, apply lanolin or vaseline twice a day. If vaseline is used, make certain that it is rubbed in well. Wipe off any surplus vaseline with cotton wool.
(ii) If the nipples have become cracked, bathe them three times a day in a solution made from ½ teaspoon (3 ml) boracic acid added to ½ pint (250 ml) water. After bathing, dry the nipples gently but thoroughly with cotton wool and apply lanolin or vaseline.

Prevention
The nails of puppies should be filed once a week.

121 Nosebleed (Epistaxis)

Nosebleeds are symptoms and the dog owner should be more concerned with the cause than with the nosebleed itself. In most instances a nosebleed will stop of its own accord fairly quickly.

Causes
Nosebleeds can be the result of:
Car accidents
A sharp blow
Tumours
Decayed tooth sockets
Excessive sneezing
Foreign bodies in the nose
High blood pressure
Minute parasites in the nose

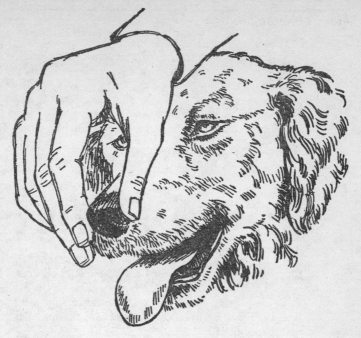

Treatment

(i) The nostrils should be sponged dry with cotton wool.

(ii) Get a good light and carefully examine the nostrils to see if the cause or site of the haemorrhage is visible. If your dog is calm and has been well trained, you should be able to do this yourself; otherwise you may need an assistant (see **Restraint**). If you can see the foreign body and if the dog remains calm, you may be able to remove it with tweezers. If you cannot see anything, do not poke about in the animal's nostrils. The mucous membrane, which lines the nostrils, is very sensitive and easily injured.

(iii) If the cause of the nosebleed is not visible, then keep the dog as still as possible. Apply cold compresses or ice cubes to the bridge of the nose.

(iv) Do not stuff or pack the nostrils. This will just make the dog sneeze and make the bleeding worse.

Tip of the nose

Bleeding from the tip of the nose can be both persistent and, if too much blood is lost, potentially dangerous. It can be controlled by pressure with the fingers (see illustration).

122   Nursing

If your dog is suffering from a severe or debilitating disease and is too weak and too sick to groom and feed itself, the nursing and loving care it receives from you will have a vital effect upon recovery. This nursing care extends to grooming and hygiene as well as to proper feeding.

(i)   Keep sick dogs in a warm, quiet, dimly lit place. Try not to disturb them.

(ii)   Keep sick dogs clean. Special care should be taken if they are suffering from diarrhoea or vomiting, for psychological as well as sanitary reasons. All animals are fastidious and become distressed if allowed to foul themselves. If they have fouled themselves, they should be gently washed with soap and water. A little talcum powder dusted on after washing is helpful.

(iii)   Larger dogs, if too weak to move themselves, should be turned regularly, every four hours, to avoid bedsores.

(iv)   Apart from doing what is necessary for its well-being, you should leave a sick dog alone as much as possible. There is a difference between loving care and fussing. Do not fuss over a sick dog.

Diet

Sick dogs and dogs recuperating from an illness need nourishing food even if they do not always want it.

Supplement their diet with a mixture of 4 tablespoons (100 ml) glucose to 1 pint (500 ml) water, daily, to supply extra energy. Do not give this, or any fluids, to a dog that is vomiting (see **Excessive Drinking**).

If the dog does have an appetite, do not give the animal all that it wants at one time. Rather, feed it smaller amounts at frequent intervals.

If the dog has no appetite, try to tempt it with strong-smelling foods such as kippers, cheese, chicken, fish, smoked salmon, tinned sardines. A dog's sense of smell, if properly enticed, will often start it eating again.

Home-made meat extracts often do the trick. These extracts are made by mincing raw meat as finely as possible and then pouring boiling water over the minced meat. The resulting liquid is then poured into a bowl, with a pinch of salt and a pinch of monosodium glutamate added to bring out the flavour.

Make every effort to tempt the dog to eat voluntarily. If nothing works, you will have to force-feed. This is a last resort. Remember, the smallest amount of food taken voluntarily will do more than a much larger amount which has been forced down.

Hygiene
All bowls, dishes, spoons, etc that come in contact with the dog must be sterilized in boiling water after each meal.

Scrupulous hygiene is absolutely essential to successful nursing.

Nursing Diabetic Dogs
See **Diabetes**. The diabetic dog requires a diet which is high in protein and low in carbohydrates. Fortunately, most canned animal foods are of this composition and provide adequate nourishment when supplemented with two raw eggs per week. Mix the raw eggs into the dog's food to provide the necessary amount of fat. Do not give biscuits or cereals.

Nursing Elderly Dogs
Elderly dogs present special problems and their general condition can be greatly improved simply by feeding them good-quality foods, in proper amounts (see **Diet**).

When nursing an older dog, whose appetite may be sluggish, stimulate the appetite by feeding meat extracts and flavourings. Since a dog's sense of smell and taste diminishes with age, some extra attention to diet will be necessary to keep the sick elderly animal eating.

Most elderly dogs are nephritic, that is, they suffer from kidney problems, and they should be fed a low-protein diet, composed of white meat (rabbit, fish or chicken), with carbohydrates in the form of rice or biscuit meal mixed in. Supplement the dog's diet with tablets of Vitamin A and Vitamin B-12, which are found in Abidec drops and Cytacon tablets respectively (available from chemists).

Elderly dogs should be given all the water they require; be sure the dog's drinking dish is always full.

Nursing Young Dogs (from birth to six months)
Diet is of paramount importance in the successful nursing of younger dogs. When dogs develop infections, their food intake falls. This is particularly dangerous with pups, which are very dependent upon daily nutrition. When they stop eating,

they begin a cycle of malnutrition and further infection, ultimately ending in death.

A young dog, weighing 2 lb (0·9 kg), requires at least 8 teaspoons (40 ml) water daily. In addition he needs a diet containing minerals, protein, carbohydrates, fats and vitamins (see **Diet**).

As long as there is no diarrhoea or vomiting, add powdered cow's milk, at twice the strength recommended for human babies, to the puppy's diet.

For puppies, Lactol is a complete diet. Feed every two hours for the first week, day and night; afterwards, every three hours for ten days. (See **Diet: Puppies.**)

If there is diarrhoea or vomiting, then neither milk nor milk products should be given. With diarrhoea or vomiting, withhold all food for twelve hours, then make a mixture of ½ pint (250 ml) water, 3 tablespoons glucose powder, 1 raw egg white, 1 pinch salt. Give 2 tablespoons every two hours. Small portions of boned chicken or fish may be given three or four times a day for four days.

If, after twenty-four hours, the puppy still refuses to eat, force-feed it with Brands Essence until food is voluntarily taken. Continue the water and glucose mixture as well, force-feeding it if necessary. If in any doubt, contact your vet.

---

123 Opening a Dog's Mouth

There are two ways of opening a dog's mouth:
(i) With your left hand placed far back on the dog's muzzle, thumb on one side of the muzzle, other fingers on the other side, you hold the dog's head. Then place the index finger of your right hand on the lower incisor teeth and prise open the dog's mouth.
(ii) With smaller dogs, the one-handed method is simply to grip the muzzle as far back as you can, and with your thumb on one side and the other fingers on the other side, press firmly on the hinge of the jaws.

---

124 Orphan Puppies

See also **Inability to give Milk.**

Very young puppies (up to four weeks old) without a mother, or those from a mother unable to feed them, should be placed in a small warm box and fed on a substitute milk supplement (such as Lactol) every two hours for the first two weeks (day and night) and after that fed every three hours.

After each feeding, they should be burped by having their abdomens rubbed gently with an oiled finger. This burping is normally accompanied by urination and defaecation.

Home-made milk supplement

If commercial substitutes are not available, you can make your own milk supplement consisting of:

30 oz (850 g) cow's milk
1 egg yolk
1 pinch bone-meal
1 pinch citric acid

Stir the mixture. Keep it in the refrigerator and then warm it to 100°F (37°C) before feeding.

Feeding technique

(i) Use an eyedropper or doll's feeding bottle. Be sure to thoroughly clean and then boil the dropper or doll's bottle after each feeding.

(ii) The amount of food required will vary with the size of the puppy. Generally, they should be fed according to their appetites. Unfortunately, some puppies have appetites larger than their capacity.

Diarrhoea

Overfeeding may result in diarrhoea. Should this develop, withhold all milk supplement and give the puppy lukewarm boiled water with glucose added – 3 tablespoons glucose powder to 1 pint (500 ml) boiled water – for two feedings. If the diarrhoea stops, return to the milk supplement.

If the diarrhoea persists for more than twenty-four hours, call a vet. If the diarrhoea was not caused by overfeeding, then it may be the result of an infection.

Solid foods

After three weeks, pups will show interest in more adult food. Encourage this new appetite by feeding them bits of boned chicken, fish and minced meat.

Weaning
Weaning, which means taking the young puppies off their mother's milk or off the milk supplement, should be complete by the time the puppy is four to five weeks old.

125 Pain

Symptoms
There is no register of pain. The owner must observe his dog's reactions as a guide to the location and severity of the pain. Dogs show pain by assuming abnormal positions or by abnormal behaviour.

Pain in different parts of the body produces different reactions. For example:

Pain in the legs causes lameness.

Pain in the abdomen causes restlessness, sitting or lying in abnormal positions, and whining. There is also a tendency to seek out cold places, such as cement floors, to lie on.

Pain in the head causes languor or restlessness, or both alternately. The dog paws at its head. The dog presses its head against the wall.

Acute pain causes the dog to cry, whine, whimper and act frightened.

The dog will look at or lick the affected area.

A dog manifesting symptoms of pain should be carefully observed for a moment. Its behaviour may give you a clue to the problem.

For example, a dog with a foreign body in its paw will chew at its foot, while a dog with a foreign body in its mouth will paw at its mouth.

After locating the site of the pain, examine it carefully with the aid of a good light. Do not let your dog's pain panic you. If you can observe and trace its cause, you may be able to alleviate it.

126 Paint, Removal of

Technique
(i) Get some cloths and rub off all the paint you can.
(ii) Then wash small areas thoroughly with soap and water and keep rubbing with dry cloths.
(iii) Snip off patches of matted hair with scissors.

(iv) For particularly difficult patches, pour a little gin or rubbing alcohol on to the patch and then rub off with a dry cloth. Hand cleaners such as Swarfega may also be used.

WARNING
Never use paraffin, kerosene, turpentine or any of the paint solvents. They cause burns on the dog's skin.

Lead in paints
(i) Paints which contain lead are poisonous when ingested. If a dog has eaten paint with a lead base, or has licked paint off its coat, treat by giving the animal a bowl of milk with the whites of two eggs beaten into it.

If lead poisoning is suspected, do not try to induce vomiting.
(ii) If the dog is in pain, or is covered with paint, try to get it to a vet. Often a general anaesthetic is necessary and, in severe cases, intravenous fluids must be administered to combat shock.

---

127 Pleurisy

Pleurisy refers to a specific inflammation of the pleura, the membrane that surrounds the lungs and lines the walls of the chest.

Symptoms
Pleurisy produces the same symptoms as pneumonia: a high temperature, painful and difficult breathing, loss of appetite and lethargy.

Treatment
Pleurisy, like pneumonia, cannot be accurately diagnosed nor adequately treated by a non-professional.

Home treatment consists of keeping the dog warm and trying to get it to take a bit of nourishment and to drink plenty of fluids.

It must be stressed that pleurisy should be considered a serious illness, and suspicion of pleurisy warrants an immediate consultation with a vet.

128 Pneumonia

Pneumonia is an infection of the lungs.

Causes
This lung infection can be caused by viruses, bacteria or worms. Sometimes, a simple chill, if left untreated, can develop into pneumonia.

Symptoms
1 General symptoms include coughing, lethargy, dullness, high body temperature.
2 Also check the dog for bluish tinges of the mucous membranes.
3 There is a definite rattling and bubbling in the dog's chest.
4 Often the afflicted dog will lie on its breastbone, with its elbow stuck out at 45° angle. This is caused by the sore chest that accompanies pneumonia.
5 When the dog is picked up, there is further evidence of pain in its chest, because its lungs are sore and picking it up compresses the lungs and increases the soreness.

Treatment
(i) Pneumonia must be considered a serious disease and professional aid should be sought.
(ii) If a vet is not immediately available, the owner must make certain that the dog is kept warm. Wrap it in a blanket, a woolly sweater, or button a cardigan around it.
(iii) Also, be sure that the room where the dog is kept is warm, and at the same time make sure there is adequate fresh air.
(iv) Try to tempt the dog's appetite with light nourishing foods.
(v) Give plenty of fluids.

129 Poisoning

Before proceeding to more detailed information regarding symptoms and treatments for common poisons, do please realize that in most instances it is just not possible for the dog owner to accurately diagnose a specific poison from observation of symptoms alone.
The only exception is when the owner has actually seen his pet eating a particular poison.

In the majority of cases, treatment must be limited to the general procedure covering all forms of poisoning.

Symptoms of poisoning
These are so broad as to include vomiting, diarrhoea, internal haemorrhage, incoordination, twitching, convulsions, coma, unconsciousness.

A glance at this list makes it obvious that all these symptoms are also present in many other conditions. Without further evidence, it is very difficult to be certain that they are caused by poison.

However, if there are grounds to suspect that a dog has eaten a poison, and providing the dog is conscious, the first rule is to make it vomit as soon as possible, except when corrosive poisons such as acids or alkalis are suspected.

Technique for inducing vomiting
The simplest and fastest way to induce vomiting in a dog is to throw ordinary table salt into the back of its mouth. The quantity of table salt will vary depending upon the dog's size. For smaller dogs, 1 tablespoon (25 ml) salt is sufficient. For large dogs, use 3 tablespoons (75 ml) salt.

The exception to this is when acids or corrosive poisons have been ingested, in which case vomiting is not desirable. When acids or corrosive poisons are suspected, give olive oil, by mouth, up to 1 pint (500 ml) for very large dogs and proportionately less for smaller dogs.

Subsequent treatment
Subsequent treatment consists of administering the proper antidote (providing you can identify the poison) and treating any symptoms as they arise.

Otherwise, administer what is hopefully known as the 'universal antidote'.

Universal antidote
When the type of poison is not known, administer a universal antidote, consisting of:

2 parts charcoal (burnt toast)
1 part magnesium oxide (milk of magnesia)
1 part tannic acid (strong tea)
1 tablespoon (25 ml) of this mixture per 20 lb (9·10 kg) *body weight.*

General note

If possible, always bring a sample of the suspected poison and a sample of the dog's vomit to the vet along with the patient. If the poison can be quickly determined, much valuable time can be saved.

If the dog is unconscious

(i) Get it to a vet. *Do not induce vomiting.*

(ii) Make sure the tongue is out. Prop open the dog's jaw with a cotton reel.

If the dog was in physical contact with toxic or corrosive substances

Wash the affected area clean with liberal amounts of clean water. Do not use soap.

If the dog is hyperexcited or having convulsions

Protect the animal from hurting itself by following the procedure for Fits and Convulsions.

If there is poison on the skin

If a poison has contacted the skin or hair, bathe the affected portions with soap and water. Even if the poison does not burn the skin, it must be removed immediately, otherwise the dog will lick its coat and ingest the poison.

Acid Poisoning

Common acid poisons are sulphuric acid (found in defoliants and car batteries); nitric acid; hydrochloric acid (spirits of salt, drain cleaners).

Symptoms

1 Inflamed patches on the skin; when the dog licks them, this leads to:

2 Burning of the mouth, demonstrated by the dog's pawing violently at its mouth and by profuse dribbling of saliva.

3 Vomiting.

Treatment for acid poisoning

(i) Administer up to 6 tablespoons (150 ml) of a solution made by adding 2 tablespoons (50 ml) sodium bicarbonate to 1 pint (500 ml) water.

(ii) Force-feed egg whites and milk. See **Force-Feeding.**

(iii) Then force-feed up to 1 pint (500 ml) olive oil for very

large dogs and proportionately less for smaller dogs.
(iv)   Get the animal to a vet.

Treatment for acid burns
Bathe the inflamed patches with a solution of 4 tablespoons
(100 ml) sodium bicarbonate to 1 pint (500 ml) water.

Alkali Poisoning
Common alkali poisons are caustic soda; caustic potash; very
large amounts of sodium bicarbonate and sodium carbonate.

Treatment for alkali poisoning
(i)   Give by mouth 2 tablespoons (50 ml) of a solution made
by adding 2 tablespoons (50 ml) vinegar to 1 pint (500 ml)
water.
(ii)   Wash the mouth out with vinegar.
(iii)   Get professional help.

Treatment for alkali burns
(i)   Apply vinegar to alkali burns by pouring it directly over
the burn, or by saturating a rag with vinegar and applying
the rag to the burns.
(ii)   Get professional help.

WARNING
Do not administer emetics or attempt to induce vomiting.

Arsenic Poisoning
Sources
Rat and mouse poisons; ant poisons; insecticides; sheep and
cattle dips; chemicals often found around smelting works and
mines. Arsenic is also a common impurity found in many
chemicals.

Symptoms
Acute arsenic poisoning may lead to death so quickly that
there is no time to observe symptoms. Smaller doses of
arsenic produce symptoms which include intense abdominal
pain; vomiting; staggering; diarrhoea; collapse; coma and
finally death. The breath of a dog suffering from arsenic
poisoning will have a strong smell of garlic.

Treatment
If the animal is conscious:

(i)   Induce vomiting.

(ii)   Force-feed the dog a solution made by adding 2 table-spoons (50 ml) bicarbonate of soda to 1 pint (500 ml) water. See **Force-Feeding.**

(iii)   Give the animal an enema of warm soapy water. See **Enema.**

(iv)   Administer demulcents – substances which cover the irritated stomach lining – such as glycerine and water, or barley water, available at chemists.

Insulin Poisoning
Usually occurs within an hour after treatment.

Cause
Diabetic dogs receiving insulin treatment at home may be inadvertently overdosed.

Symptoms
These vary from staggering and incoordination to unconsciousness.

Treatment
(i)   If the dog is still conscious, give it one to ten lumps of sugar, depending on the size of the animal (1 lump of sugar = $\frac{1}{2}$ teaspoon powdered sugar).

(ii)   If the dog has lost consciousness, and a vet is not immediately available, mix water and sugar in the amounts given above. Crush the sugar lumps between spoons to make the sugar dissolve faster, and pour a little at a time into the dog's mouth. Take great care not to choke the unconscious dog with the mixture. Hold the dog upright. See **Force-Feeding.**

Mercury Poisoning
Sources
Antiseptics and fungicides, broken thermometers and barometers.

Symptoms
Early symptoms are vomiting and diarrhoea.

If death does not occur immediately from shock, the early symptoms are followed by ulceration of the mouth and tongue, then acute kidney failure.

Treatment

The absorption of mercury into the system is very rapid and swift treatment is essential.

If the dog's stomach can be emptied within half an hour of ingestion there is a good chance of recovery.

(i) Induce vomiting by throwing a tablespoon of salt into the back of the dog's mouth.

(ii) Force-feed egg whites and milk (2 egg whites to ½ pint (250 ml) milk). See **Force-Feeding.**

(iii) Then induce vomiting again.

Phosphorus Poisoning
Sources

Unspent matches, rat and mouse poisons, cockroach poisons, the striking surfaces of matchboxes, fireworks.

Symptoms

1 The classic symptoms of staggering, abdominal pain and vomiting are present. But if phosphorus poisoning is suspected, pay particular attention to the vomit, which will glow in the dark. The dog's breath and vomit will have a strong odour of garlic.

2 Following the onset of these symptoms, there is a period of apparent recovery, which may last from three to four hours to several days.

3 This recovery period then ends, and the abdominal pain and vomiting recur, together with jaundice – a yellowish tinge appearing in the eyes and mucous membranes – and nervous symptoms which if ignored will lead to coma and death.

Treatment

Treatment must not be delayed. The specific antidotes for phosphorus poisoning are given below in (ii) and (iv), but if these are not available, administer the Universal Antidote (see above).

(i) At the first suspicion of phosphorus poisoning, induce vomiting by throwing a spoonful of salt into the back of the dog's mouth.

(ii) After causing the dog to vomit, force-feed a solution of 1 teaspoon (5 ml) of 1 per cent copper sulphate to 1 pint (500 ml) water. See **Force-Feeding.**

(iii) Induce vomiting again.

(iv) Then administer 1 teaspoon (5 ml) potassium permanganate in 1 pint (500 ml) water.

(v)   Give the dog an enema of warm soapy water. See **Enema.**

(vi)   Do not give any fats in the dog's food for the next five days.

Strychnine Poisoning

Sources

Rat, mouse and mole poisons.

Symptoms

The first symptoms of strychnine poisoning are excessive nervousness, restlessness, noticeable twitching of the muscles, and stiffness of the neck.

As the condition progresses, these symptoms become more pronounced and convulsions suddenly occur.

In convulsions caused by strychnine poisoning, the limbs are extended and the neck is curved upwards and backwards.

During the early stages, these convulsions are sporadic, but they will become progressively more frequent, until any external stimulus – the slightest touch or noise, even a current of air – will produce them.

During this later stage, the pupil is widely dilated, covering nearly the whole surface of the eyeball.

Finally, death is caused by the inability to breathe, due to paralysis of the respiratory muscles.

Treatment

(i)   If the dog is having convulsions, it must be anaesthetized by a vet. Do not try to take the dog to a vet. You will not make it. Have the vet come to the dog.

(ii)   If convulsions have not begun, induce vomiting.

(iii)   After vomiting, force-feed the dog up to 1 pint (500 ml) strong cold tea (tannic acid). See **Force-Feeding.**

(iv)   Further treatment must be left to the vet.

(v)   While waiting for the vet, it is important to keep the dog very quiet and insulated from any external stimuli which may trigger off these convulsions. Place the dog in a quiet darkened room.

---

130   Post-Puerperal Metritis

This condition causes an abnormal vaginal discharge that

occurs shortly after the bitch has given birth.

Symptoms

1 Two to five days after giving birth, there is a heavy, dark, bloody discharge from the vagina.

This discharge should not be confused with the slight, greenish-brown discharge which is normal after a bitch has had a litter.

2 Increased thirst.

3 High temperature. (The normal discharge is not accompanied by high temperature and greatly increased thirst.)

4 Dullness, depression.

Treatment

Treatment must be given by a veterinary surgeon. The above symptoms merit his immediate attention.

---

131   Poultices

Use

The prolonged application of heat to a swelling or to a sore area will relieve the pain and control the swelling.

The advantage of a poultice is that it retains its heat without having to be constantly changed.

There are several types of poultice but the simplest and one of the most effective is a kaolin poultice.

Kaolin is a china clay from Cornwall and is available in tins, from all chemists.

The poultice is prepared by heating the tin in a saucepan full of boiling water. When the clay is fairly hot, it is spread on a bandage and this bandage is then taped over the affected area.

Before placing the bandage on the dog, test a bit of the kaolin on the back of your hand. It should be very warm, but not hot enough to cause you any pain.

The poultice should be changed every four hours.

Substitutes

If kaolin is unobtainable, poultices may be made from bread or from potatoes.

To make a poultice from bread, boil some water, soak the bread in the boiling water, allow it to cool enough for you to handle it, then apply it to the affected area.

To make a poultice from potatoes, simply mash some cooked potatoes and apply them to the affected area.

132   Prolapse of the Rectum

One of those conditions that look much worse than they really are.

Actually, it is fairly common in puppies suffering from persistent diarrhoea. Occasionally, it is seen in older dogs as well.

Treatment
(i)   Wash your hands.
(ii)   Gently wash the area around the anus with warm soapy water.
(iii)   Apply liquid paraffin liberally around the anal area.
(iv)   Gently push back the protruding portion until the anus is normal.
(v)   Wash your hands again.

133   Prostatitis (Enlarged Prostate Gland)

The prostate gland is found only in the male animal.

Causes
Old age, hypersexuality.

Symptoms
Difficulty and obvious pain in passing motions. Passage of flattened or ribbon faeces.

Treatment
Problems with the prostate gland can be serious and require professional treatment. Antibiotics and possibly female hormones may be indicated.

If a vet is not immediately available, administer liquid paraffin (1–3 tablespoons (25–75 ml), depending on the size of the dog) to enable the dog to pass a motion with less difficulty. (See also **Constipation.**)

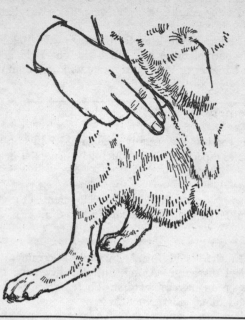

134 Pulse Rates, Respiration Rates and Average Rectal Temperature

Normal pulse rate for dogs   80–120
Average rectal temperature for dogs   101·3°F (38°C)

As a general rule, the smaller the breed or species, the higher the pulse rate.

135 Pulse Taking

See illustration.

Technique
Place your index and middle fingers over the femoral artery at the point where it crosses the thigh bone on the inside of the thigh, almost in the groin.

Count the pulse beats for one minute.

The smaller the dog, the faster the pulse rate, which, depending upon size and individual animal, varies from eighty to ninety beats a minute when the dog is in good health.

In a dog running a high fever, the pulse rate may be as fast as 160 beats a minute.

The important thing for the dog owner to know is his own pet's normal pulse rate when the dog is in good health, so that a higher or lower pulse rate will not go unnoticed.

136 Pyometra

This condition is usually seen in older (five to six years old) females especially those which have irregular heat periods.

Cause
A pus-producing, abnormal development of the cells lining the womb. The condition occurs in two forms:

Symptoms
1 In the 'open form', there is a creamy, foul-smelling, vaginal discharge. Along with the discharge the bitch will develop an increased thirst. There will also be some degree of abdominal enlargement.

However, pyometra is not an infectious disease, so there will not be any dramatic rise in body temperature.
2 In the 'closed form', there is no visible sign of a discharge.

The reason is that in this form the bitch's cervix remains closed and the uterus gradually fills up with pus. This produces a pronounced enlargement of the abdomen, extreme lethargy and increased thirst.

Treatment
Both forms of pyometra must be considered serious, and they require surgical treatment. Consult a vet immediately.

137 Restraint: The Handling of Dogs

By restraint we mean the technique of handling, moving and holding a dog largely against its will.

When to use restraint
When one must do something which the dog finds frightening, painful or objectionable.

It is never pleasant to use restraint but when it is necessary, be firm, unhurried and know what you are going to do *before* you approach the dog.

There are several methods of restraining reluctant dogs. The method you use depends upon:

1 The size of the dog
2 Your purpose in restraining the dog. Do you want to move the animal or to hold it?

Techniques

(i) The first step in restraining a dog is to make sure that it does not bite you. The easiest way to do this is to tape its mouth closed.

(ii) Take a bandage or necktie, wrap it around the dog's nose, knot it, and then tie the free ends around its neck, behind the ears.

(iii) The dog may then be held by your putting an arm around its neck. With your other arm, hold the dog around the hips. Hold the animal against your body to prevent it from wriggling out of your arms.

Small dogs

Small dogs or those with short noses are more difficult to restrain, but they can be handled by having a rolled towel wrapped around their necks (see illustration).

A variation of this technique is to get behind the dog, grab the scruff of its neck with one hand and grab its back legs with your other hand and stretch them.

Large dogs

Get behind the dog, grab it firmly by the skin of the neck, just behind the head, with one hand on one side of the head and the other hand on the other side. The dog may now be either held or dragged.

138 Rickets

Symptoms

Rickets affect young dogs from three weeks to six months old. The first sign is usually a noticeable swelling of the wrist joint. Swellings will also be observed running along the side of the chest.

Severe cases will eventually develop bending of the long leg bones, causing bow-leggedness.

(i) General method of restraint

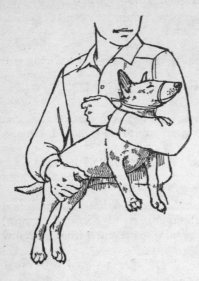

(ii) First method of restraining a small dog

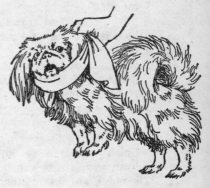

(iii) Second method of restraining a small dog

(iv) Restraining a large dog

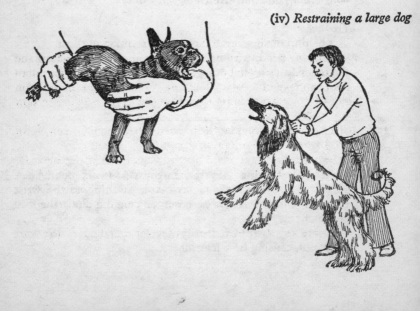

Causes

Rickets are the result of a calcium, phosphorus and Vitamin D deficiency.

Treatment

(i)   Mix sterilized bone-flour into the dog's food. (1-4 teaspoons per day).

(ii)   Give Abidec drops: two to three drops daily.

(iii)   Administration of cod-liver oil is not recommended for young dogs suffering from rickets, since cod-liver oil can alter the calcium to phosphorus ratio in the bones if given in excess of two drops daily.

---

139   Ringworm

Ringworm is a disease of the top layer of the skin (epidermis) caused by two groups of fungi, *both of which are contagious and infectious, and can affect human beings.*

Ringworm is rare in dogs and easily confused with other skin diseases, such as demodectic mange.

Symptoms

Breaks in the skin appear on the head and chest. These are dry scaly patches, circular in shape, up to 1 in (2·5 cm) in diameter. These lesions vary from very slight to scaling of the skin, followed by a pus-forming infection.

Treatment

(i)   Clip the hair around the breaks in the skin.

(ii)   Apply a dilute solution of Cetavlon to the lesions and the surrounding area (solution: 1 teaspoon (5 ml) Cetavlon to 10 teaspoons (50 ml) water). Saturate cotton wool in the solution and continue application for as long as the breaks in the skin are visible.

(iii)   The specific and most successful treatment for ringworm is the oral administration of griseofulvin tablets.

In healthy dogs, the condition will disappear spontaneously, in about two months. But do not wait two months, because in addition to being contagious, ringworm is a highly unpleasant and very uncomfortable disease and it should be treated at the first sign.

(iv)   Always wash your hands after treatment of a dog with ringworm.

140   Saline Solution

A sterile (germ-free) salt solution, used to wash eyes, wounds, etc.

(i)   Dissolve 1 teaspoon (5 ml) block or cooking salt (iodine-free salt) in 1 pint (500 ml) boiling water.
(ii)   Allow the water to cool to body temperature, then apply.

141   Sebaceous Cyst

Cause
Blockage of the duct of a sweat gland.

Description
These cysts are found on the dog's skin, usually on its back. They often have a pustular head and resemble a miniature volcano.

Treatment
If you leave the cyst alone, it will usually rise to a head and eventually pop, discharging a cheesy substance.

When the cyst does pop, it should be thoroughly squeezed out. The area around the cyst should be bathed with a dilute solution of antiseptic Cetavlon and water. Use 1 teaspoon (5 ml) Cetavlon to 10 teaspoons (50 ml) water.

Occasionally, a sebaceous cyst will rise to a head, pop and continue to discharge without healing. If the cyst does not stop discharging, it will require surgical removal.

142   Sedative Overdose

Sedatives, in the form of sleeping pills, are often left around by careless owners and eaten by unwary pets.

Symptoms
1   The dog will stagger about and appear very drowsy. It will keep trying to go to sleep.
2   There may not be an empty pill container to confirm your suspicions. The dog may have eaten it along with the pills.

Treatment
(i). Contact a vet immediately.
(ii) Induce vomiting.
(iii) Administer stimulants. Strong tea or black coffee, cooled, should also be given.
(iv) Keep the dog awake. Walk, drag, if necessary, the dog around. Keep the animal walking until the effects wear off.
(v) If the dog keeps falling asleep, slap its face to keep it awake.

143 Shampooing a Dog

(i) Wet the dog down thoroughly.
(ii) Lather a good-quality hand soap or mild shampoo into the dog's coat.
(iii) Wash all the lather out of the dog's coat.
(iv) Be careful not to get any soap in the dog's eyes, or you will find it twice as difficult the next time you try to give the animal a bath.

Contrary to a widely held belief, this frequent washing does not remove the oils from the coat; rather, it stimulates production of these natural oils. If skin conditions are present, use a selenium-based shampoo, such as Selsun.

In addition to monthly baths, dogs should be given a good brushing every day.

The long-haired breeds should be combed as well as brushed to prevent tangling.

144 Shock

Shock is the term used to describe a state of collapse which is characterized by an acute and progressive failure of the circulatory system.

Causes
While the exact causes of shock are unknown, the condition follows most forms of severe injury, massive haemorrhages, heart failure, serious burns and dehydration.

Symptoms
(Following severe trauma, ie serious accidents): Apathy; low body temperature; pale gums and pale tongue; a rapid thready

pulse; rapid shallow breathing; thirst; and, finally, complete collapse.

Treatment
(i) First aid treatment consists of keeping the dog warm by wrapping it in a blanket. Then allow it complete rest. Keep the dog quiet and get it to a vet.
(ii) The prime form of treatment is to restore the amount of circulating fluid in the blood-vessels through a transfusion, which can be administered only by a vet.

---

145 Sinusitis

Sinusitis is an infection of the sinuses. (The sinuses are an extension of the nasal chamber, located in the front of the head.)

Causes
The infection may be caused either by germs or by a foreign body in the nose.

Symptoms
Except in the case of foreign bodies, sinusitis rarely occurs on its own. It usually is seen as a sequel to virus conditions such as *distemper*.

The symptoms themselves are:
1 A yellowish nasal discharge.
2 Bouts of sneezing.
3 Loss of appetite.

Treatment
Since many other illnesses are characterized by the same symptoms, you will need professional help to make a definite diagnosis. So, if the symptoms continue for more than twenty-four hours, take the dog to a vet. (If it is sinusitis, the vet will probably administer a course of antibiotics.)

If a vet is not immediately available, home treatment consists of:
(i) Keeping the dog's face clean of the mucous discharge, and
(ii) Assisting the dog to breathe normally by clearing the nasal passages.
This is accomplished by inhalations of a preparation of friar's balsam or menthol in hot water. To make this preparation,

place some boiling water in a large, shallow tin dish (a pie tin) and add 3 tablespoons friar's balsam or menthol to the boiling water. Then, calmly but firmly, hold the dog's face over the steam for a moment or two.

Try to treat this inhalation as an ordinary occurrence. The trick is to have the dog inhale as much of the vapour as possible; and this is only effective if the dog is not alarmed.

Also, you do not want to hold a struggling frightened dog over boiling water, so do not force your pet, just handle the animal with confidence.

---

146 Skin Diseases: General

Dogs can develop acute skin conditions very quickly. These conditions are very painful and very unhealthy and should not be allowed to continue. Prompt treatment by the dog owner can prevent nuisances from becoming serious problems.

The most obvious indication of skin problems is excessive scratching. Any dog that is continually scratching itself either has trouble or is heading for trouble. The owner must take note of this scratching and set about discovering its cause.

Also, skin diseases have a public health aspect. Some, such as ringworm and sarcoptic mange, can be transmitted from animals to people. Others, eg demodectic mange, are transmitted from animal to animal.

Skin diseases take various forms and many factors are involved, but for purposes of home treatment, we can divide skin diseases into:

1 Contagious (which means it is transmitted by direct contact).
2 Infectious (which means it can be transmitted through the air), eg ringworm.
3 Non-contagious, such as eczema and hormonal imbalance.

Contagious and infectious
These diseases, as well as fleas, lice, mange mites, and ringworm should be treated under strict hygienic conditions, and the affected dog should be kept away from other animals and from small children.

Non-contagious
With the non-contagious skin diseases the owner may not feel the same urgency for treatment. Some owners, in time, even get used to their dog's condition and 'learn to live with it'.

These owners would do better to learn to cure it.

Aside from eventual worsening of the original complaint, neglect invites a host of secondary complications.

All abnormal skin conditions should be diagnosed and treated at once.

Among the forms in the non-contagious category of skin diseases, perhaps the most common is warts. These may be due to viruses, but this has not been proved.

If the owner will take his pet to a veterinary surgeon when he *first* observes this growth, it is usually simple to remove. But the longer the owner waits, the more difficult and the more dangerous the operation becomes.

Hormonal imbalance

This is a common cause of non-contagious skin disease. The imbalance can produce hairlessness as well as certain varieties of eczema. If the symptoms are observed and treatment instituted early on, the condition can be quickly corrected.

Hereditary diseases

Owners of highly bred dogs, especially those bred for certain abnormal traits such as the folds and protruding eyes of the bulldog and the squashed nose of the Peke, should be aware of the particular skin diseases their animal's breeding makes it heir to (see **Breed Failings**).

Neuroses

Highly-strung dogs and dogs which need a lot of exercise and are not getting it, or dogs which are simply neurotic (yes, there are such creatures) may develop skin diseases by continuously licking themselves. Usually they pick out a spot on their foreleg and just lick it until the skin breaks.

Treatment

(i) Apply calamine lotion to the affected spot.
(ii) If the dog continues to chew and lick at it, it may be necessary to bandage the area.
(iii) An Elizabethan collar may be necessary.

External origins

Chemicals, accidents, foreign bodies (such as grass seeds), even overexposure to light, can cause a skin disease.

Allergies

Probably the most common of non-contagious skin diseases

are those caused by allergies. Unfortunately, they are also the most difficult to cure.

147 Slipped Disc

This painful condition of the spine is fairly common in dogs with long bodies and short legs, such as dachshunds and corgis, but instances of it do occur in all breeds.

Causes
Breed failing, obesity. Also occurs in dogs which are violently overexercised.

Symptoms
Acute pain, especially when the dog attempts to walk. In severe cases, the dog cannot move its legs.

There may be rigidity or tenseness of the abdomen. Touch the dog's stomach lightly. The skin will be as tight as a drum.

There may be retention of urine and faeces, at first. Then, as the bladder and small intestine fill up, the animal is unable to control itself and there is involuntary passage of the body wastes.

Treatment
The first thing to do is to ease the dog's pain. Administer one 300 mg aspirin tablet for small dogs, up to 1500 mg for large dogs, once every twenty-four hours. See **Tablets and Pills: Techniques of Administration.**

The severity of the symptoms indicates the severity of the condition and while most mild instances of a slipped disc will right themselves, a vet should be consulted.

If the condition persists or recurs frequently, surgery may be necessary.

148 Sneezing

Continual sneezing is a much more serious symptom in dogs than in humans.

Intermittent sneezing
If the dog sneezes on and off for a few hours, but otherwise seems all right – no temperature, no apathy, etc – the cause of

the sneezing is probably due to simple irritation, such as dust up the nose.

Prolonged sneezing

If the dog continues to sneeze throughout the day, refuses food, and there is an accompanying nasal discharge, suspect an infection and get professional assistance.

Bursts of strenuous sneezing

Strenuous and continued sneezing suggests a *foreign body in the nose*.

Examine the nostrils. You will need a good light for this. (An electric torch is ideal.)

If the foreign object is visible, use tweezers and carefully remove it.

WARNING

If you do not see anything, do not poke about with your tweezers. The nasal lining is easily ruptured (see **Nosebleed**).

---

149   Sprains and Strains

Sprains and strains are very similar in their effects and symptoms. A *sprain* involves the ligaments around a joint. A *strain* involves muscles. In both cases, the tissues are torn.

Causes

Sprains and strains are usually caused by violent exercise.

Symptoms

The diagnosis must often be made as the result of negative findings for fractures and dislocations. After these have been eliminated as the cause of the dog's lameness, look for a slight swelling around the joint or muscle.

Treatment

(i) Alternate hot and cold compresses over the swelling until it goes down.

(ii) If the animal is very uncomfortable, administer an analgesic.

150   Stains at the corner of the Eye

Certain breeds, especially the poodle, may develop brown staining at the corner of the eye.

Cause
Blockage of or absence of tear ducts, leading to weeping (epiphora).

Treatment
Make a very dilute solution of 20 vol hydrogen peroxide – 1 teaspoon (5 ml) hydrogen peroxide to 10 teaspoons (50 ml) water – and bathe the stains liberally. *Do not bathe the eyeball, just the stains.* This not only gets rid of the stains, but in the case of blockage of the tear ducts, it may also remove the obstruction.

151   Stings

Treatment
If you have seen an insect sting your dog, try to locate the sting, which will be at the top of the swelling, and remove it by pinching at the bottom of the swelling with a pair of tweezers or a couple of wooden matchsticks. Only a bee sting is left behind.

Do not try to pull out the sting with your fingers. You will only succeed in making matters worse by squeezing the balance of the sting's contents into your dog.

Bee stings
Washing soda should be applied directly on the bite. This will relieve the pain of the bee sting.

Wasp stings
For wasp stings, use vinegar, applied directly over the bite.

For bites in the mouth, use an ice pack to reduce the swelling.

Should the swelling or swellings, in the event of multiple bites, become very large (golf-ball size or larger), or if the dog has difficulty in breathing, get the animal to a vet immediately. This is an emergency.

In these severe cases, if a vet is not available, try an animal-loving doctor, dentist or even a pharmacist. An injection of antihistamine is necessary.

Dosage
The dosage varies with the particular antihistamine used. With Piriton, 4 mg will be sufficient for a small dog (see **Body Weight of Dogs**).

Mild cases
Fortunately, most stings are not so severe and the pain usually subsides after half an hour.

For mild discomfort, lasting longer than half an hour, administer aspirin. See **Analgesics**.

---

152 Swallowing Safety Pins or other sharp Foreign Objects

Feed the dog bread or porridge. Also feed it small balls of cotton wool, which have been dipped in meat extract, such as Bovril, for flavouring.

Avoid force-feeding.

---

153 Swelling of the Abdomen

A sudden and dramatic increase in the size of the abdomen suggests:
1 Overeating.
2 Pregnancy.
3 Tumours.
4 Fluid in the abdomen as a result of liver or heart failure.
5 Pyometra.
6 An ovarian cyst.
7 Enlargement of the liver.
8 Enlargement of the spleen.
9 Torsion of the stomach.

---

154 Swelling of the Eye (Glaucoma)

Causes
This condition is caused by failure of the fluid of the eye to circulate. Often a breed failing. Seen in wire-haired fox terriers and Bull terriers cocker spaniels and Bassets.

Symptoms
The eyeball increases in size and protrudes from the eye socket.

There is usually associated conjunctivitis and, in later stages, corneal opacity (a cloudiness of the front of the eye).

Treatment
Glaucoma, like all eye conditions, must not be treated by a non-professional. A vet will administer drugs to improve the circulation of fluid. The only thing the dog owner can do is get the dog to the vet.

---

155   Tablets and Pills: Techniques of Administration

Concealment
If the dog is not being starved, conceal the pill or tablet in a tasty titbit such as meat, cheese or soft-centred chocolate.

However, some dogs are notorious for finding even the most cunningly concealed pill. In this case, be prepared to administer the pill directly.

Direct technique
(i)   Place your left hand on top of the dog's head, with your thumb and index finger placed behind the canine teeth.
(ii)   Pull the dog's head upwards.
(iii)   The tablet is in your right hand. Use this hand to open the dog's mouth by holding the lower jaw behind the lower canine teeth.
(iv)   Push the tablet as far down the dog's throat as possible.
(v)   Hold the dog's jaw shut.

---

156   Taking Samples of Faeces and Urine

Technique
To assist your vet in diagnosing certain illnesses, a specimen of the animal's faeces or urine will be needed.

Since dogs do not always 'perform' at the most convenient time and place, this may require some persistence on the owner's part.

The best time to collect the sample is first thing in the morning.

Collect the sample of faeces immediately and put it in a tin or can, clearly labelled with the dog's name, the dog owner's name and address, and the date.

Collecting a sample of urine requires even more persistence.

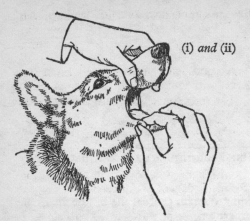

(i) *and* (ii)

(iii) *and* (iv)

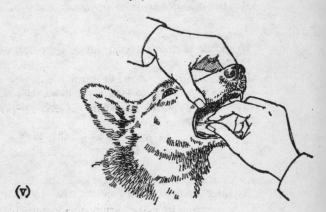

(v)

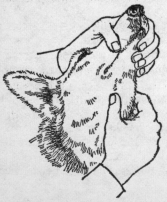

Do not try to collect the sample directly from the dog into a bottle.

Use a sheet of polythene, shaped with a dent in the centre. Let the dog smell the polythene sheet before it urinates, so that it will not be too alarmed when you try to catch the urine in it.

A saucer or scallop shell may also be used, but you will have to be very quick.

As soon as the dog begins to pass water, place the polythene sheet in the best position to catch the urine, and then transfer it to a clean bottle. Make sure the bottle is clearly labelled.

Fortunately, one does not need a great deal of urine for laboratory analysis. A few drops will be sufficient.

---

157 Tar on the Feet

An occasional nuisance for owners of adventurous dogs.

Treatment
(i)   Stand the dog in a basin full of warm salt water with olive oil added.
(ii)   Whatever tar does not wash off during the foot bath should come off when you dry the dog's feet with a rag.
(iii)   If all the tar does not come off after the first washing and drying, repeat the process.

---

158 Tartar on the Teeth

Causes
All dogs living in a hard-water area eventually develop tartar on their teeth.

Symptoms
1   Bad breath (halitosis).
2   The dog, while obviously hungry, either refuses to eat, or begins to eat, then spits out the food. There is usually excessive salivation and pawing and rubbing at the mouth.
Should these symptoms occur, examine your dog's teeth. Tartar looks like brown crusts on the teeth.

Treatment
(i)   In the early stages, tartar can be rubbed off with smoker's

tooth powder. Remember, tartar accumulates on the back of the teeth as well as on the front.

(ii)   In particularly stubborn cases, professional scaling by a veterinary surgeon may be necessary.

Prevention
Prevention of tartar accumulation can be accomplished by regular (about once a month) cleaning of the dog's teeth with either ordinary toothpaste on cotton wool, or with smoker's tooth powder on moist cotton wool.

---

159   Teething Stages in Puppies

Like humans, dogs have two sets of teeth. The temporary teeth (or baby teeth) appear about three weeks after birth. These are replaced by the permanent teeth which appear from five months onward. As the permanent teeth push through the gums, they displace the temporary teeth which are either spat out or swallowed. By the sixth or seventh month, all the permanent teeth are in.

Dogs have twenty-eight temporary teeth and forty-two permanent teeth.

Complications
The temporary canine teeth often remain in the dog's mouth after the secondary or permanent teeth have appeared. These extra teeth may have to be extracted when the dog is six to eight months old. (This condition is particularly common in the smaller breeds, especially the Yorkie and the poodle).

Care of teeth
(i)   Dogs should have regular dental checkups, by a veterinary surgeon, to prevent gingivitis, periodontitis, halitosis and eventual tooth loss.

(ii)   The wise owner will accustom his dog to having its teeth cleaned regularly with toothpaste (or else with a mild abrasive cleaning powder on cotton wool).

---

160   Temperature Taking

Most infectious and contagious diseases in the early stages cause the body temperature to rise. This rise in body temperature is often, but not always, accompanied by lethargy and loss of appetite. Identification of temperature and its severity provides the dog owner with a guide as to whether a vet should be consulted.

Taking a dog's temperature is not at all difficult. The technique is very simple.

Type of thermometer
Any stubby, bulbed clinical thermometer may be used. Such thermometers are available at all chemists.

Technique for taking a dog's temperature
A dog's temperature must always be taken by rectum. (If you put a thermometer in a dog's mouth, the animal will probably try to eat it.)

(i)   Have someone hold the dog while you take the temperature. (If there is a possibility that the dog might bite, tape its muzzle (see **Restraint**); but a well-trained pet should allow its owner to take its temperature without making too much of a fuss.)

(ii)   Hold the thermometer by the end opposite the bulb, between your index finger and thumb, and then shake it with a sharp jerky movement until the mercury is down to 95°F (35°C). When you first do this, it is best to do it over a thick rug or bed, so that if you do drop the thermometer, it will not break.

(iii)   Dip the bulb of the thermometer in some vaseline, cold cream or baby oil.

(iv)   Approach the dog from the rear, and gently slide an inch of the thermometer through the anal sphincter, using a gentle rotary action. Be prepared to stop the dog from trying to sit down.

(v)   Push the thermometer in with a light touch, letting it find its own direction.

(vi)   Once the thermometer is in place, support the protruding end very lightly and wait one full minute.

(vii)   Then withdraw the thermometer, wipe it clean with cotton wool or Kleenex and read the temperature.

Reading a thermometer
(i)   All clinical thermometers are marked in degrees, with large marks and small marks for each $\frac{1}{5}$ degree.

(ii)   After withdrawing the thermometer from your dog, hold it up to the light and, still holding it by the end opposite the bulb, roll it between your fingers until you see the silver band of mercury.

(iii)   Calculate the degree of temperature.

Chart of normal body temperature
Dogs: 101·3°F (38°C)

A temperature of 102·5°F (39°C) and higher is significant and good reason to consult a vet.

When calculating temperatures, remember that an excited or frightened dog has a higher body temperature than a relaxed one; so subtract a degree or two if this is the case.

When you have finished using the thermometer, wash it in *cold* water. If you use the same thermometer on more than one animal, dip it into alcohol, to prevent the transferring of bacteria.

Should the thermometer break while in the dog, take the dog to a vet, if possible. If a vet is not available administer liquid paraffin (not kerosene): 1 tablespoon (25 ml) liquid paraffin orally, three times a day, until the thermometer is expelled with faeces.

---

161   Ticks

Country animals quite often come into contact with the common sheep tick. Usually, ticks are first noticed when you are grooming your dog: another good reason for frequent grooming.

Description
The tick is a blood-sucking parasite with a shiny spherical body, varying in size from ¼ to ½ in (0·5 to 1 cm) in diameter. The tick is creamy-grey in colour. It looks something like a soya bean with tiny legs at one end.

Treatment
Do not try to pull the tick out. Ticks have powerful sucking jaws which are imbedded in the dog's skin. If you try to pull the tick out, its head will break off, leaving the mouth of the tick under the dog's skin, and a sinus may eventually form. (A sinus is a discharging wound that does not heal.) The trick is to get the tick to remove its mouth *before* you pull it off your dog. There are three techniques for accomplishing this:

(i)   Pour a little ether or petrol-lighter fuel on to a pad of cotton wool, and then place the pad over the tick, for half a minute. Then pull the tick out.

(ii)   Smear each individual tick with vaseline and then remove it with tweezers.

(iii)   Hold the lighted end of a cigarette very close to the tick, without actually touching it or the dog. The heat will make the tick withdraw its head, and it may then be removed.

If the head of the tick does break off, clean the skin around the area with Cetavlon, or soap and water.

Using a boiled (sterile) needle, remove the head of the tick from under your pet's skin exactly as you would remove a splinter from your own finger.

In areas where ticks are common, bathe the dog in a solution of ·06 per cent benzene hexachloride, every three weeks. (This is available from chemists.)

---

162   Tonsillitis; Choking; Foreign Bodies in the Throat

These three conditions produce similar symptoms.

General symptoms

1   The dog will cough, lick its lips, appear distressed and may cry out in pain. It will refuse food and may appear apathetic or sleepy.

2   Bones stuck between the larynx and the stomach cause no loss of appetite, but when the dog eats, it vomits. Also, there is excessive dribbling and the dog will be profoundly depressed. There is no home treatment for bones lodged in this area. Professional treatment is necessary.

Treatment (foreign body in the throat or mouth)

(i)   First, open the dog's mouth. Using an electric torch, look down its throat.

(ii)   If there is a foreign body such as a bone stuck in the dog's throat, use your fingers or, if it is too far down to reach, a pair of pliers, to ease it out gently.

Symptoms of tonsillitis

1   The dog will appear to be choking.

2   When you open the dog's mouth, the tonsils, which are

at the back of the throat, will look like two swollen, strawberry-coloured lumps.

3 The dog will be very depressed.

4 The dog will have a high fever: temperature over 103°F (40°C).

5 It may vomit.

6 It may cough.

Treatment of tonsillitis

(i) Calm the dog with petting and soothing words. Then administer one or two 300 mg aspirin tablets per day, depending on the size of the dog.

(ii) Give no food or water, except for some cracked ice, until a vet has examined the dog.

(iii) Put the ice into a perforated bowl (a soap dish with holes punched into it is ideal), so that the dog can moisten its mouth by licking the ice but cannot drink.

---

163 Tourniquets

The purpose of a tourniquet is to stop the flow of blood from a severed artery or vein.

In an emergency a tourniquet can be improvised from many things: a necktie, belt, strip of material, shoe-lace; even a strip of plaited grass will serve.

If the dog is bleeding badly, try to staunch the bleeding so that you can observe the way the blood is flowing: this indicates whether the dog is bleeding from an artery or a vein.

Arterial wounds

If the blood comes out in a pumping fashion in time with the heartbeat, and is bright red, then it is from an artery and the bleeding must be stopped quickly or the dog will die.

For arterial wounds (on the limbs) make a tourniquet by wrapping a bandage or belt around the limb, *above* the injury. Then insert a pencil or screwdriver into the bandage, and twist the tourniquet until the bleeding stops.

Venous wounds

Blood flowing from a vein flows regularly, rather than being pumped out. The colour is dark red.

For venous wounds, apply the tourniquet *below* the wound, and twist until the bleeding stops.

Keep the tourniquet tight for no more than one minute. Then loosen slightly.

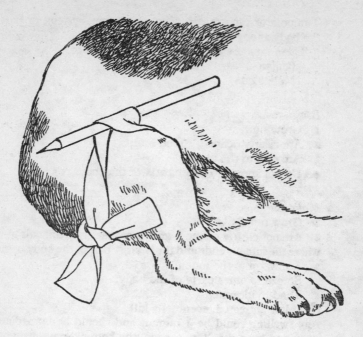

Every ten minutes, loosen the tourniquet completely to see if the bleeding has stopped, and to allow the blood to reach the rest of the leg and prevent tissue damage.

164 Trembling or Shivering

Causes

Dogs shiver when they are:
1 Frightened.
2 Cold.
3 Running a high fever.
4 Excited.

Shivering or trembling that goes on for longer than half an hour is a sign that something is seriously amiss.

Examine the dog for fever.

165   Tumours

Tumours or cancers can affect any organ, system, or part of the body at any age.

These tumours are divided into two groups:
   Benign
   Malignant

Benign tumours
1 Grow slowly.
2 Are clearly defined, round lumps.
3 Are cool to the touch.
4 Do not spread to other parts of the body.

Malignant tumours
1 Grow rapidly.
2 Are not clearly defined, and it is sometimes difficult to tell where the tumour ends and the healthy part of the body begins.
3 Are warm to the touch.
4 Spread to other parts of the body.
5 Tend to ulcerate.
6 If left untreated, eventually kill.

Any swelling could be a tumour and should be immediately examined by a vet. The sooner, the better. Some malignant tumours can be stopped if they are caught early enough.

166   Unconsciousness

When you find a dog unconscious, unless the cause is immediately apparent, such as a great gaping chest wound, do not waste time looking for the cause. The only exception to this is when the animal has been in contact with an electric wire (see **Electric Shock**).

Just because the dog does not appear to be breathing, do not assume that it is dead, unless certain other factors are valid. Even if you think the dog is dead, and though you cannot detect breathing, give artificial respiration for at least thirty minutes.

The reasons why animals lose consciousness may be divided into two very general categories: primary and secondary causes.

Primary causes

The dog loses consciousness as the result of a lesion affecting the nervous system and brain. This occurs after car accidents or similar injuries, fits, strokes and narcosis produced by poisoning.

Secondary causes

The dog loses consciousness as the result of causes affecting other areas of the body.

These include diabetic coma; uraemic coma (poison from the kidneys); calcium deficiency; shock; electric shock; drowning; and heart attack.

Fainting, causes of

Dogs faint if the blood supply to the brain is reduced or when it is deficient in oxygen. This occurs in dogs which are in a state of shock, or whose hearts are not functioning properly.

Treatment

Dogs that have fainted will recover spontaneously.

Make sure the animal's tongue is out and that nothing is blocking the windpipe. Most dogs recover from faints in three or four minutes.

167 Urethral Obstructions; Bladder Stones (Cystic Calculi)

The urethra is the tube running from the bladder to the outside of the dog. On occasion, this tube becomes irritated or, in severe cases, blocked.

Symptoms

Inability to pass urine; distended abdomen; standing in a peculiar, splay-legged position; and a profound depression and apathy.

Cause

Depending upon the seriousness of the symptoms, this condition could be caused by anything from a mild cystitis infection, to bladder stones, to complete blockage of the urethra. Blockage of the urethra is serious and must be treated without delay.

EMERGENCY
If your dog displays these symptoms, this is an emergency. You must have professional help immediately. Do not attempt to prod the distended abdomen or the bladder may rupture. If this happens, the dog will die.

168 Vaccination

Definition
A vaccine is an injection of either living or dead viruses, that provide immunity to certain virus diseases.

Natural immunity
Puppies receive antibodies from the first mother's milk, which is called colostrum. This provides a natural immunity which lasts for eight to ten weeks and then diminishes.

In order not to interfere with this natural immunity, puppies are usually not vaccinated until they are ten weeks old.

Orphan puppies
Orphan puppies which are being fed on supplements and not receiving colostrum, should be given an injection (by a vet) of gamma globulin, when they are two days old. They should be vaccinated at eight weeks and again at twelve weeks of age to insure a high immunity against distemper and hepatitis.

Dog vaccines
A single combination vaccine is available to prevent distemper (hard pad), hepatitis and the two types of leptospirosis.

169 Vomiting, Causes of

1 Infectious disease, eg distemper.
2 Acute abdomen, eg peritonitis, intestinal obstruction.
3 Indigestion, eg overeating.
4 Metabolic disorders, eg hepatitis or nephritis.
5 Drugs, eg digitalis.
6 Nervous problems, eg motion sickness, fear.
7 Pharyngeal irritation, eg tonsillitis.
8 Poisoning.
9 Parasites.

10 Hernias.
11 Tumours.
12 Inflammation of the gullet (oesophagus).
13 Tonsilitis.
14 Toxaemia.

---

170 Warts

Description

Small, pinkish, rounded lumps on the dog's skin. Most frequently found around the muzzle and the top of the head.

The cause is not definitely known, but warts may be caused by a virus. In any case, they are not serious, and since they will not trouble your dog, do not let them trouble you.

Treatment

Warts which have a definite neck may be removed by dog owners. Tie the wart off with a piece of cotton. In two or three days, the wart will drop off.

Otherwise, warts are easily removed by a veterinary surgeon.

---

171 Weaning

Weaning is the process of taking a puppy off its mother's milk and putting it on to a diet of more adult food.

Puppies begin showing an interest in solid foods at three or four weeks old. This interest, however, does not mean that they are quite ready to be weaned. But their interest should be encouraged by offering them small amounts of finely chopped minced meat, boned fish or chicken, and bowls of milk, three or four times a day.

When the puppies are six to seven weeks old they are ready to be weaned.

By the time the mother begins vomiting her food (soft, partially digested) for her youngsters to eat, they should be completely weaned.

At about eight weeks of age, recently weaned puppies should be given five meals a day: three of meat and two of cereal (that is, fine puppy meal, cornflakes or Farex mixed with milk). (See **Diet for Younger Dogs**.)

If you wish, commercial dry food preparations may be given. With dry foods, feed up to five times a day, depending upon the brand.

172   Weight

Increase in Weight
A great increase in weight over a short period suggests
1   Compulsive eating, which may be the result of simple greed or brain damage. This compulsive eating is also seen in dogs which have been desexed.
2   Abdominal tumours.
3   Pancreatic tumours.
4   General tumours.
5   Fluid in the abdomen: renal, cardiac, or hepatic.

Treatment
A definite diagnosis and treatment must be given by a vet. The above list is only a guide to the possible causes of a sudden increase in weight.

Loss of Weight
Sudden loss in weight may be caused by:
1   Reduced intake of food.
2   Persistent vomiting.
3   Reduced absorption of food due to a disease such as chronic nephritis, or hepatitis.
4   Diabetes mellitus.

Treatment
Try to identify the cause, then treat the symptoms as they arise. In the event of continuing weight loss, get professional assistance.

173   Worms

Worms are one of several types of parasite which may try to use your dog as their host.

Unpleasant as they are, worms rarely cause serious problems, except in puppies. During the first eight months of the dog's life, the owner should be alert to the possibility of worms.

Causes
The worms are picked up from other animals and from the faeces of affected animals.

Symptoms
Worms in young dogs produce a variety of symptoms. These may be seen separately or in association with each other.
1 Vomiting of worms.
2 Worms in the faeces.
3 A pot-belly.
4 Halitosis.
5 Failure to grow correctly.

Adult symptoms
In adult dogs, the presence of worms is rarely detected until the worms are either coughed up or appear in the faeces.

WARNING
While most types of worms are not particularly dangerous to the dog itself, the round worm can be transmitted to humans and may cause blindness.

One more good reason why children should not be encouraged to let stray puppies lick their faces. And a good reason for insisting that they wash their hands before eating, after playing with *any* animals, including their own.

Obviously, the differential between diagnosis of hook worm, whip worm, round worm, etc cannot be made by the dog owner. Therefore, it is advisable to treat all worms and suspected worm conditions with hygienic precautions.

Treatment
For worms other than tapeworm, administer piperazine tablets (available from chemists), 500 mg per 10 lb (4·5 kg) *body weight*. Repeat in one week.

Tapeworms
Symptoms
1 Tapeworms rarely cause any severe or dramatic symptoms, apart from a change in the texture and colour of the coat.
2 There may be some non-specific illness and diarrhoea. By 'non-specific' illness we mean that the dog may be off form: nothing specific, nothing you can put your finger on, just not well.
3 The observant owner will notice segments of tapeworms in the faeces, and other segments of tapeworms sticking to the hair around the anus.

Description

The dog owner will have no difficulty in distinguishing the tapeworms. Indeed, it would be difficult not to distinguish them.

When freshly passed, these segments are about $\frac{1}{4}$ in (0·5 cm) long, moist and quite active.

They dry rapidly and shrivel up. When dry, they resemble small, brownish grains of rice.

These dried-up tapeworms are often found in the dog's bedding.

Treatment

Fortunately, treatment is simple and usually effective. There are a number of excellent commercial tapeworm preparations available, eg Dichlorophen. Administer 500 mg per 6 lb (2·7 kg) *body weight*, after a meal. Then wait seven days and repeat the dose.

Since the tapeworm is carried by the flea, get rid of the fleas as well as the tapeworms. See **Fleas.**

---

174   Wounds

A wound is a break or 'lesion' of the body surfaces. When the wound occurs, the dog bleeds. If the wound is superficial and the bleeding slight, in the normal course of things the blood will clot and the bleeding will stop. But if the dog is losing a lot of blood, first aid must be administered.

Treatment

The first priority is to stop the bleeding, irrespective of whether or not it is arterial or venous.

(i)   If the dog is bleeding very badly, do not waste time. Jam a wad of rags, Kleenex or a towel over the wound. Press hard and hold it there until the bleeding stops. If nothing else is available, use your hand or fingers pressed directly on to the wound to stop the bleeding.

(ii)   Once you have staunched the wound, try to determine whether it is arterial or venous.

If the blood is bright red and spurting, it comes from a severed artery. If the blood is deeper red and oozing, it comes from a vein.

(iii)   For arterial wounds, apply a tourniquet between the wound and the heart.

(iv) For venous wounds, the tourniquet is applied on the side of the wound farthest from the heart.

(v) If the wound is on the trunk, or on the neck, where a tourniquet cannot be used, you will have to keep pressing the wad of material or your hand over the wound until the bleeding stops. When you do remove the pressure, be careful not to tear away the protective clotting and start the wound bleeding again.

(vi) Once the bleeding has been controlled, the next step depends upon the severity of the injury and whether or not the dog is in a state of shock. If it is, then it must be treated for shock. If not, proceed to treat the wound.

Dressing the wound
(i) Clip the hair around the wound with blunt-pointed scissors.

(ii) Wash the wound with soap (any good-quality hand soap) and cooled boiled water. If you have an antiseptic such as Cetavlon or Dettol handy, use it. Otherwise, just soap and water will do. Be sure to wash away the dirt, oil, or grease from the centre of the wound.

(iii) After drying, apply a simple dressing to keep out infection. A pad of cotton secured with elastoplast will do the job. Change the dressing once a day.

(iv) For severe wounds, after cleaning and dressing, administer *antibiotics*.

The most efficacious treatment for a wound can be deduced from observing the type of wound it is.

Classification of wounds
1 Clean incised wounds. These bleed freely and a pressure bandage or tourniquet should be applied.
2 Lacerated wounds. These are jagged irregular wounds, which bleed minimally and require ordinary bandaging.
3 Puncture wounds are usually the result of bites and are nearly always infected.
4 When accompanied by bruising, wounds are known as contused wounds.

Chest Wounds
Treatment
Place a moistened pad or wad of material directly over the wound.

If there are any plastic bags or sheets of polythene available, place them over the pad and hold them in position with elastoplast or ordinary sticky tape to obtain an airtight shield over the wound.

In an emergency, do not waste time looking for a pad or wad of material. Use your hand or fingers to stop the bleeding. Put your hand or fingers directly on the bleeding wound, and press. This should stop the bleeding until you can get a proper dressing on it.

Do not remove the dressing.

If a wound continues to bleed through a dressing, apply another pad and bandage it tighter, or apply more pressure by hand over the wound. Do not remove the first dressings. This will only disturb the blood clot which is forming over the wound and make the bleeding worse.

Transporting a dog with a chest wound
(i) Move a wounded dog only when you must.
(ii) If you can hear air sucking in and out of the wound carry the dog with its breastbone down, otherwise carry the animal with the wound uppermost.